Early Book Reviews

"You have taken putting soap in the mouth for naughty words ..." to a New Level! LOL Who knew we were surrounded by so many toxins.

I've pretty much finished your book now working on giving sections to my family and friend that I think will especially appreciate certain chapters! YOU my Dear have found your calling, YOU make this rather "dull" subject a Very Good, interesting read, with fun personal touches along the way.

I LOVE your book; I hope people will embrace it. Why worry so much about health care if we keep killing ourselves with poison. We can all start with eliminating the toxins out of our lives.

Val Peterson

It Feels Good To Feel Good

Learn to eliminate toxins, reverse inflammation and feel great again

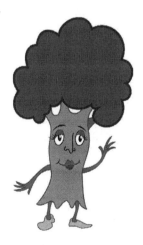

Cheryl Meyer

Illustrations by Nicholas Patton

It Feels Good to Feel Good
Learn to Eliminate Toxins, Reduce Inflammation and Feel Great Again.

For permission requests, email the publisher or author at
cheryl@cherylmhealthmuse.com
or send your request to

122 E Walnut Suite A
Monrovia, CA 91016

To contact the publisher, visit
Cherylmhealthmuse.com

To contact the author, visit
cheryl@cherylmhealthmuse.com
ISBN-13: 978-0692827284 (Custom Universal)
ISBN-10: 0692827285

Library of Congress Control Number: 2017906325
Cheryl Meyer, Monrovia, CA

Printed in the United States of America

For information, contact Cheryl Meyer at cheryl@cherylmhealthmuse.com

The content of this book is for general informational purposes only. It is not meant to be used, nor should it be used, to diagnose or treat any medical condition or to replace the services of your physician or other healthcare provider. The advice and strategies contained in the book may not be suitable for all readers. Please consult your healthcare provider for any questions that you may have about your own medical situation. Neither the author, publisher, IIN nor any of their employees or representatives guarantees the accuracy of information in this book or its usefulness to a particular reader, nor are they responsible for any damage or negative consequence that may result from any treatment, action taken, or inaction by any person reading or following the information in this book.

Table of Contents

It Feels Good To Feel Good

Learn to eliminate toxins, reverse inflammation and feel great again

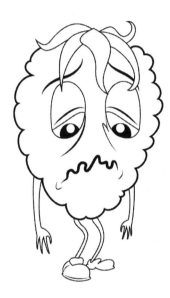

Dedication

This book is dedicated to people with pain and inflammation. It is also dedicated to people who want to raise healthy families and are unaware of all of the toxins in our world. It is dedicated to all of the people struggling with any of the 100+ autoimmune diseases.

How to use this book

There are hundreds of suggestions in this book to help you purge toxins out of your life and your immediate environment. I have purged these toxins from my life; however, I did accomplish this over a 5-year period. It could take you 5 years to do all of this. You can't do it all at once, and you will be frustrated if you even attempt it.

I suggest you take a yellow highlighter as you read this book, and highlight the things that would be easy for you to do first.

Doing all of this will be a process and you will take little steps every day until they are all accomplished. Celebrate each win. Do not beat yourself up if you slip, or think you are removing the toxins too slowly. Every step you take will bring you closer to wellness. Work at a comfortable pace for you. **If you email me at cherylmhealthmuse@gmail.com, I will send you an eBook workbook to use to take notes.** I will help you stay on track.

THE TOP STRATEGIES TO USE THIS INFORMATION

There is a full index.

1. Read the book and get informed

    It all starts with information and awareness. I was stunned when I began to discover how many toxins were in my life. Get on email lists for the people recommended in my Part 6, Chapter 28 *Amazing people who are leading the way taking on the system*. Information changes and is updated regularly. Stay informed.

    Support the organizations in Part 6 Chapter 27 *Organizations to Follow and Support*. Get on their Facebook and email lists. The work these dedicated people are doing, on all of our behalf, is worth following, learning from, and supporting.

2. Get a yellow highlighter pen

   As you start to read, highlight the things that would be easy for you to do right away. Once you finish the book, make a list. This is where to start. You can go through the book again later to implement more things.

3. Start with food.

   - Before you eat anything, ask yourself *"what nutrients are you feeding your body by eating that food."* If there is no food value, don't eat it. Period. Eat to nourish your body. Stop eating processed food. Stop eating fast food. They contribute absolutely nothing for your body to utilize.
   - **COOK.** It's the only way you can control what you are eating. If you haven't been cooking, start simple and easy. It doesn't have to take more time than eating fast food. It just takes a little planning and having the right ingredients on hand. THIS IS THE MOST IMPORTANT CHANGE IN EATING THAT YOU CAN MAKE IN YOUR LIFE AND THE LIVES OF YOUR FAMILY. Crowd out bad food choices by having great food choices on hand.
   - Enjoy sitting around the table at dinner and sharing your day with each other. The joy and love of community is an important step to health.
   - Use the *Dirty Dozen* and *Clean 15* charts included from **EWG, the Environmental Working Group**. Always buy organic if the item is on the *Dirty Dozen* list. Eventually you will want to buy all organic, but for now start there.
   - Familiarize yourself with ingredients that are genetically modified. (GMO) Avoid them. You don't need these toxins in your body.
   - Add more vegetables and fruits to your diet. Eat from all of the colors of the rainbow; each has a gift of nutrients that determine the color.
   - If possible, buy local. The closer you are to your vegetable being grown and coming to market, the more prime the nutrients are.
   - Get tested for your food sensitivities, and eliminate anything on your list. This is a biggie to eliminating inflammation and pain.
   - Adopt a "Do This, Not That" strategy. When you read a recipe, see what ingredients you can swap to make a healthier version of it. Be creative. Have fun. This is a get-well journey. I find it both fun and rewarding to

creatively change an unhealthy recipe, to one that is now both yummy and healthy.

Start thinking about food hacks. If you have always used white wheat flour, try almond flour instead. If you have always used low-fat or non-fat (skim) milk, try whole milk. Try organic dairy. Try raw dairy. Or learn to use alternative milks, coconut milk, almond milk, cashew milk. If the recipe calls for "bad" cooking oil, substitute the oil for ghee, or coconut or avocado oil. If it has sugar, cut the quantity by 2/3 and add a little stevia. Use coconut sugar, or maple syrup or raw honey, but only enough to add a little sweetness. (Sugar is sugar is sugar.) Avoid fructose, corn syrup and white sugar. At least honey, coconut sugar and maple syrup have some trace minerals that are good for you. Keep swapping until everything you eat and feed your family is a healthier version. Do this over time. Experiment.

- Cut out a major portion of simple carbohydrates from your diet. If it's white, it's processed and not good for you. (White flour, white sugar, white rice.) Drastically reduce the sugar in your diet. It's as addictive as cocaine, and it is harming all of your body functions. It is triggering inflammation.
- Stop using fake sugar chemicals. The pink, blue and yellow packets should be thrown away. Swap them for Stevia (without additional chemicals) or honey or maple syrup in a limited quantity. Remember, sugar is sugar is sugar, so drastically reduce the amount but stop eating the chemicals.
- Think "Pegan"[2] if you choose to eat meat. ¾ of your plate should be vegetables. Meat becomes a condiment on your diet. It's much easier to afford pastured organic meat if you eat smaller portions of it. You still get all the benefits.
- Read food labels.
    - If there are things you cannot pronounce, they are chemicals. Don't buy it.
    - Look at the order of the ingredients. If a sugar is in the top 5, pass.
    - Look at how many grams of sugar are in each portion. 4 grams of sugar = 1 teaspoon

- ○ Pay attention to portion size. There are often 2 or more portions in a container.
- ○ Buy GMO free. Look for **GMO Verified** on the label. You don't need the pesticides and herbicides in your body.
- ○ Look for canned goods that are BPA free.

4. If you aren't getting the answers you need for your health from your doctor, find another practitioner. I recommend a Functional[3] or Integrative MD. There are lots of things you need a conventional MD for – like heart disease, or kidney problems. Own your health, no matter what type of doctor you are working with, keep pushing for answers. You will find them. You aren't crazy and there are solutions.

5. Engage your entire family in your wellness journey. Do not isolate one sick member. Everyone in the family can benefit from your new wellness strategy. Educate and inform them as you learn. Put a plan together. You will all be more successful if everyone is enrolled in their health. You will raise healthier children.

6. Do not even attempt to throw out all of your family's favorite foods. Find healthier substitutions first. As you run out of a food, swap it for a healthier version. (I.e. Chemical cereal with tons of sugar, for oatmeal, or organic brown rice crispies, or Cream of Buckwheat.) Watch out for chemicals and high sugar and swap them for low chemicals or no chemicals and low sugar.

7. Plan ahead. Plan what you need before you grocery shop. Having healthy ingredients on hand leads you to making healthy meals. Plan healthy choices to take with you when you are out and about. Always have healthy protein bars (low sugar, high fiber, no ingredients you can't pronounce) in your purse or in your car if you are hungry. Don't be in a position of making bad food choices because you didn't plan ahead. This is actually very easy to do and you will thank yourself.

8. Investigate restaurants before you go out to eat. Call ahead, and engage them in what they can prepare for you so that you can eat healthy there. You will be surprised at how accommodating they will be.

9. If you find yourself in a situation where the good food choices are limited, eat one of your protein bars, and a green salad and some vegetables on the

menu, and enjoy the company of the people that you are with. Find joy in the company you are with, not in the heavy chemically laden foods they are eating.

Most important, DON'T PREACH. You will find plenty of resistance from your family, your friends, and your co-workers. They will clean up their world when they are ready. Lead by example. And, don't let them convince you to go back to bad food choices. Stay the course.

OTHER THINGS YOU CAN BEGIN TO ADOPT RIGHT AWAY

1. When you run out of a cosmetic, replace it with a healthier choice
2. When you run out of a cleaning product you use, replace it with a healthier choice
3. Get a filter on your kitchen sink and drink water that has fewer chemicals. Find a non-plastic container so that you can take your own filtered water with you when you are out of the house. (I use stainless steel)
4. Limit the over the counter drugs that you use. Try one of my drug swaps. They work.
5. Get 7 hours of sleep each night
6. Work on your primary elements. You need to take care of you, before you can take care of everyone else. You are worth it.
7. Confront toxic relationships, and make them healthier or set boundaries
8. Adopt a stress reducing strategy; start to do the 4-7-8 breathing exercise. It takes a couple of minutes, and works miracles.
9. Move. You can take a walk, or try one of my suggestions. But you need to move, so do something.
10. Become an "army of one." Get involved. Vote with your dollars. We can change the system if we put our money where our health is.

This is a fraction of what you can change but even this is a hefty "to do" list. There is no timetable to accomplish all of this. Each step you take is one step closer to a pain-free, joyous life. Celebrate with each win. Congratulate yourself for the progress you are making. Be grateful that you have a chance to impact your health little by little. Make it fun, for you and for your family.

And **KEEP GOING**. You will learn how great it is, to feel good again, and it will all be worth it.

It Feels Good To Feel Good

Learn how to eliminate toxins, reverse inflammation and feel great again

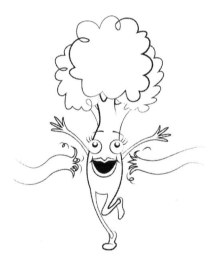

Who am I, and why did I decide to write this book?

My name is Cheryl Meyer, and I recently became a Health Coach. (Cheryl M Health Muse) I am certified through the HCTP program at the Institute for Integrative Nutrition®.

I am writing this book to help others who have pain from inflammation. I want to share what I have learned in the process of eliminating my own pain.

I got sick, really sick five years ago, and I was saddled with pain.

I got sick because I was not paying attention to how I was eating and I was ignoring my body. And, to boot, I had oodles of toxic lifestyle habits.

- I was not listening to my body.
- I had an ostrich approach of not paying attention to the available information that could have helped me.
- I took no time to take care of myself, or even notice what my body was saying or feeling.
- I was busy taking care of everyone else, my staff, my mom, my friends. It's a lovely thing to be a caretaker, but I had to learn that I also had to take care of myself.
- I was eating on the fly, or going out to dinner often eating rich, heavy food.
- I was eating late at night.
- I was rarely cooking.
- I gained a lot of weight.
- I was working 24/7.
- I was feeding on stress.
- I was in a love relationship that had turned toxic.

And ... I didn't understand why organic was important or what damage GMO's (genetically modified foods, defined in Part 3, Chapter 6) and toxins were doing to my body.

Unaware that all the pre-signs and circumstances for sickness were in place, the pain began.

I did not recognize the early signs of inflammation and didn't understand what was happening to my body. However, I was aware of the increasing pain in my body. I often woke in the middle of the night in pain. When I woke up in the morning, I could barely get out of bed. It was painful to move, and sections of my body hurt. My brain was confetti. My moods were all over the place.

My MD took a conventional approach that wasn't helping me. In all honesty, I think she didn't know how to help me. And I was resistant to taking additional pills.

I knew I needed to lose weight, but I didn't want to diet, and I didn't want to change the way that I ate. It seemed that changing what I ate would lead to a life of deprivation.

So, it was Pain with a capital P that set me on a five-year journey to get well and to make drastic lifestyle changes.

"You change, when you get sick and tired of being sick and tired."

UNKNOWN

My significant other broke up with me. More pain.

Since my conventional doctor was no help, I started looking for a medical practitioner that could help me. Little did I know that unless I was in a diseased state, conventional medicine didn't want to tackle my symptoms like low cortisol or a slightly off thyroid. My medical tests showed results out of range but not diseased. Therefore, my conventional MD didn't perceive these results to be an issue because I wasn't in a "diseased state." In my case, I later learned that conventional medicine was not even running the correct tests to find the problem and that also may be true for you. My doctor certainly didn't know where to go digging for the source of my pain. And she expressed that it was "all in my head" and to take 2 Aleve.

The only solution offered for my pain was drugs.

I went to the "leading expert" on autoimmune disease in Southern California, another conventional MD, but this time a specialist. Since I didn't have all of the symptoms of any of the commonly known autoimmune diseases, he also didn't perceive that I had an issue. All my symptoms combined were an odd sized peg that didn't fit into a round hole. Therefore, in his mind, it couldn't be autoimmune. He offered me steroids. When I refused, he too told me to take two Aleve a day. Again, he had been trained to assess the symptoms and prescribe the pill.

My conventional doctor missed that I had Type II Diabetes. I had to push her to test me. I had dealt with Hypoglycemia as a young adult and knew something could be wrong with my blood sugar. Little did I know that since I had had Hypoglycemia earlier in my life, it was normal to get Type II Diabetes later in life.

I found a Doctor of Chiropractic who was an integrative nutritionist. He started me on my path to eating healthy and exploring my medical tests beyond "normal." After six months, when none of the weight came off, and when the aches and pains only showed modest improvement, he announced I was a very sick girl and that he didn't know how to help me.

So, I decided to take ownership of my own health. Taking ownership was the "ah-ha" moment when my health began to turn around.

I found Functional Medicine online, and I started to listen to every Functional Medicine symposium on health issues that was available, from autoimmune to thyroid to adrenals, to gluten sensitivity. I am enormously grateful for the incredible knowledge I gained from the functional community for free. I started buying books by these experts and reading like a fiend. Most of the speakers had been very sick themselves and were renowned in their own respective fields. They were accomplishing amazing results with their patient base. They had found a way back to wellness themselves. Their approach was very different from my experience with conventional medicine, both for myself and also for my parents, where I had been very involved, but who were now deceased. See my upcoming chapter on Functional Medicine (Part 1, Chapter 3) to understand the difference in approach.

I studied toxins that might be impacting my life. I had been born with several allergies, so it made sense to me to start there. (I now understand that they were probably sensitivities. They didn't make that distinction 60 years ago. I suffered from foods that gave me rashes and made me sick. I often reacted to medications. My joke was that I popped out allergic to Pittsburgh. Whenever I got within 50 miles of Pittsburgh, I broke out in a rash from head to toe. I remember them oiling the streets to keep the coal and steel dust down. We left when I was 4.)

I had taken an **allergy** test with my conventional MD, but found I was only allergic to the tape that held the test on my back.

When I found a Functional MD that practiced "root cause" medicine, she helped me discover all kinds' imbalances that needed correcting in my body. I took a **sensitivity** test, and I found out I had severe reactions to a variety of foods from chicken to herbs and common vegetables, to dairy, to soy, and to gluten. At the time, I reacted to gluten so severely that I even reacted to meat from animals that ate grains. I removed all these foods from my life. A sensitivity test looks for different markers than an allergy test. (More about this later.)

I cut sugar out of my life and went through drug withdrawal. It felt as if I was coming off a high from cocaine, or maybe even heroin, and in fact, it was similar. Who knew? I was so sick in the beginning of the detox; it was worse than a bad flu. I was super sick and in bed for days.

I was diagnosed with Undefined Autoimmune Disease. I will offer an explanation of inflammation and autoimmune disease, next in this book, including what it is and how to heal it. This information could save your life. It is the fastest growing disease in the United States.

This information will explain to you if you hurt why you hurt, why you have gained weight, and how your body should work as an orchestrated symphony. If your adrenals are not working correctly, they impact the liver, the gut, the brain and the rest of the body; similarly, with the liver, or the pancreas, or the thyroid, etc.[6] Your gut is the second brain and impacts your entire immune system, as well as depression and Alzheimer's. Any part of your body that is off key will affect the entire performance of your body.

Finally, I will cover toxins and how they impact your body, your family, and the environment. You will begin to understand inflammation, and I will give you some of the necessary tools you will need to put out the fire.

Regaining my health has been a process, like peeling an onion. Under each layer, there are new issues to address and correct. My Functional MD and I are still finding new conditions that need to be targeted and healed. But I am no longer frustrated. We are finding answers, and looking in entirely different places to find the keys to wellness.

SIX REALIZATIONS THAT MADE THE BIGGEST DIFFERENCE TO MY PAIN:

1. The conventional MD that I was seeing wasn't helping me; I needed to own my own health to alleviate and end the pain (without steroids or over the counter drugs)

2. Pharmaceuticals weren't going to cure me. There is no magic pill. Although they can make the body "feel better" the majority of drugs do not get to the "root cause" of the ailment. Even worse, they often carry their own set of complications and side effects.

3. I needed to discover and then avoid all of my sensitivities.

4. I had to begin to eat as clean as possible (eating fewer toxins, eating live food.)

5. Toxins needed to be removed from my life as quickly as possible from all of the products I was using at that time. I started an investigation to discover what they were.

6. I found a Functional MD and a Functional Chiropractor who practiced "root cause" medicine. Because of them, and their knowledge and guidance, my pain is almost gone.

This book is mostly about these six revelations. It took me five years of research, and trial and error to clean up my food, my cosmetics, my personal care products, my cleaning products, my mind (I cleared out the *ANTs**), my stress and my toxic relationships.

These revelations made me decide that I am a primary player in healing my body and my life.

It was about learning how to pay attention to my body and to start taking care of myself.

What I recommend in this book is a lot to take on. It is a process.

This book encourages you to partner with your doctor on your quest for wellness and to become educated enough to find solutions to your own health issues. Both you and your doctor are critical players in helping you find wellness. Your health care professionals (and I have a team of functional health care professionals) will guide you through the way the body works and how to make it well. This book is a proactive guide for you to follow, outlining the things that you can do to find wellness on your own.

If you follow the advice outlined in this book, you will be well on your way to healing your pain, but I repeat, it is a process. These are all things that you can do for yourself to improve your health. I want you to do the best you can, each step of the way. Incidentally, along the way, I have lost 45 pounds; 45 pounds of toxic weight. Not from dieting, but by eating real food. I still have more weight to lose, but by eliminating all of the toxins, my body is functioning closer to how it was meant to, and my excess weight is starting to slowly fade away.

I also found a wonderful new guy who totally supports my journey, and married him two years ago.

This book is for you if:

- You are healthy and want to stay that way
- You are sick, and you hurt, have brain fog and low energy and need help cleaning up your lifestyle and eliminating your pain
- You are gaining weight
- You are puffy from inflammation
- You are taking care of a sick family member or sick child that has lots of sensitivities, or allergies, and you need guidance
- You are sick and willing to do anything you can to improve the quality of your health. (You can accomplish it without deprivation).

As your Health Muse, I will also make suggestions of things I have found that make my eating and my life quite enjoyable, in spite of the out of the norm way I am eating compared to the majority of America. No more SAD (Standard American Diet) for me, no more processed foods or fast foods or too much sugar or genetically modified grains and vegetables. These things were killing me. And I do NOT feel deprived, in any way, eating completely different from other people. In fact, by eating healthy, I feel good again. Being delightfully different from others, in this instance, has incredible benefits.

Each of us is unique, so the solutions that have worked for me may be different than what will work for you. At least I can get you started, share resources with you, and name the products that have been beneficial for me so that you have a jumping off point. If my recommendations are not right for you, I will lead you to where you can research on your own to find optimal products.

Buying organic and locally sourced foods are no costlier than buying that daily Frappuccino and fast food, especially when you are preventing costly medical bills in the long term by doing so.

My advice could save you money in other ways. I have bought dozens of products that were low in toxins, but that did not do the trick for me. After a lot of trial and error, I have been able to compile a resource list of excellent products that I have found that work, and I share many of them with you in this book. There are additional resources on my website, www.cherylmhealthmuse.com. As I discover new products, I will add them to the list on my site.

I am slowly purging all toxins out of my life, and now have excellent suggestions so that you can do the same.

I have tried a variety of eating principles and have settled on Paleo[7] [8]. But we are all different. Vegan[9], Vegetarian or Raw[10] may work for you. I have experimented with all of these approaches. The key is to start somewhere, purge the toxins, eat real food, and then listen to your body. The key is that the majority of your diet should be beautiful vegetables and fruits that give your body nutrients to live.

Some of the things I have learned along the way are downright frightening. Many of the ingredients Big Food companies are using are synthetic fake ingredients that your body can't use and have no food value; these fake ingredients are even causing your body harm and creating your pain. Your body is starving on these "foods."

What Big Chemical is doing to our Food supply in conjunction with Big Food, is poisoning us. Big Chemical is inserting many toxic chemicals into our lives, our fabrics, our cleaning supplies, and our personal care products.

We will also look at what Big Pharm is doing to cover up your ailments with drugs that are creating an entirely new list of issues and dysfunctions in your body along the way. This conversation about Big Pharma includes over the counter drugs.

It's all pretty frightening stuff. But you have the power to avoid these toxins for you and your family.

I have even learned how conventional doctors only get half a day of nutrition in medical school. Hence the general advice, you need to lose weight with absolutely no guidance as to how to do that, except to be vigilant. You know the good ole *Willpower* advice that doesn't work and makes you feel bad. Their only other advice is to exercise, which is good advice and an important part of the puzzle, but the advice they are offering is not enough to lead you back to wellness. Conventional doctors have good intentions; they just never learned a nutritional approach in medical school so they don't know how to help you.

Other things that I have learned are just down right amazing.

The body has an incredible ability to heal itself if we give it proper nutrients.

What an amazing machine this body is that we call home.

Why aren't we shouting this from the rooftops? (Because there is no money in it!)

I want to set you off in the right direction, as you begin your own journey. I want to teach you to own your own health, and then you can take it from there. But for you to "buy in" to what I am telling you, I am asking you to change your "known truths," which are often not true. These thoughts are what you have been told and accepted your entire life about doctors, about what you eat; about your food and about how you live. These outdated thoughts are still accepted by the majority of Americans.

I am asking you to believe that the world is not flat.

You can do that, right? You've <u>already</u> accepted that the world is round.

I am asking you to believe that our medical care system is broken and that there is a better way.

We are living in the dawning of a new age of health, food, and self-care that will take a bit of faith in the beginning but will serve you well the rest of your life. It is a complete paradigm shift from what we have been told is true.

If this all seems daunting, I can help you; I am a certified Health Coach, and I have been through all of this. I can inspire and guide you to find a new path where you take responsibility for your own health. Please contact me through my website. Https://cherylmhealthmuse.com. I do coaching via Skype, Facetime or any other platform that you have available to you. I also do face to face coaching in my office in Monrovia, California. I plan to start group coaching in my Monrovia office to help people return to eating real food and also help them purge the toxins. I will expand this to webinars later in 2017, so if you are interested, sign up for my mailing list on my website.

If you want to know more about me, my website is very transparent about where I have been, what I have gone through, and how I think it could help you.

The bottom line is I want to educate you to begin to heal yourself and make some drastic changes. We are a very sick nation, and there are solutions.

One of the first things said to me was:

"If you don't take care of your body, where are you planning to live?"

DR. TONY GANEM

I heard it, it resonated, and I changed.

But as I say this to others, there is resistance and confusion about the concept.

People will listen once they begin to recognize they are losing their health and they start to search for a better way.

"You will change, when you get sick and tired of being sick and tired."

UNKNOWN

This book is a guidebook of all of the self-directed things you can do now, for yourself, to impact how you feel. It's about how you can be proactive and own your health. It's about creating an environment where your children can thrive.

"No one said it was going to be easy; they just said it was going to be worth it."

UNKNOWN

It starts with education and then takes commitment to feel good for the rest of your life.

I am hoping to inspire healthy people to change now so that they don't get sick. Inflammation and Autoimmune disease begin years before the actual symptoms start to appear. The approach I want to teach you is the healthiest lifestyle you can have for long-term health, for you and for your family, no matter how you all feel now.

And I am especially encouraging people with inflammation and pain, and/or autoimmune disease to make these changes now to create a better future and reverse the inflammation.

What I am suggesting is a new way of viewing food, what you eat, and your social interactions over food. It's a significant shift in paradigm. Eventually, as a country, we all need to do this. We are a nation in a state of disease and it is getting worse. I am asking that you be a pathfinder with me, and an example for others. I assure you that your health and your body will thank you.

As I contemplated changes for myself, some resonated with me immediately. I knew they were right and that they made sense.

- It resonated that I needed to eat more live food.
- I knew I needed to eat food that was local so that the nutrients were still prime.
- I knew I needed to eliminate pesticides and herbicides from my diet and my body. (Ingesting these substances that kill bugs and funguses couldn't possibly be good for us.)

By understanding these concepts on a core level, I was able to make those changes and to incorporate them into my life fairly quickly.

Other changes I needed to make were harder to accept.

- I didn't want to be different from everyone else; I am very social, and to me, food was also community; food was love.
- I needed to see the success of this approach before I accepted it was the correct path.
- I needed to understand why it was important to eat organic. I learned, that at the very least, it is important to eat organic fruits and vegetables that are subjected to the most toxins. (The Dirty Dozen[11] list) I have also learned why it is crucial to avoid GMOs (genetically modified foods.)
- I needed to know that this approach wasn't about deprivation.

Once I did, these all became easier to do and maintain as a permanent lifestyle change. And I eat plenty of delicious food that is also nutritious. There is no deprivation in my life.

I learned that community has nothing to do with food. It has to do with enjoying the people you are with at the time, whether you are eating the same foods they are or not. I have learned that there are many kinds of food, and not all of them go into my mouth.

I am also asking you to root out all of the toxins in your life. This book is a comprehensive guide to accomplish that.

These changes are things that I stumbled upon in my journey to find wellness. I had no idea that I was living in such a toxic environment: the food I was eating was toxic, the cosmetics I was using were toxic, the cleaning products I was using were toxic, and the over the counter drugs I was taking were toxic. That even the water I was drinking was toxic.

One of the main reasons I wrote this book is because all of this information was not available in one place. It was scattered all over the place, and although all of this information can be found on the internet, I had to do quite a bit of digging to find what I needed. This was a five-year discovery period. In the beginning, I didn't even know what information I was looking for and what I needed to learn. I want to give you the advantage of learning what I have discovered all in one place. I don't know about you, but it is much easier for me to implement and sustain lifestyle changes when I understand the "why."

And now that most of the toxins are out of my life, I feel amazingly better.

All I can tell you is, it feels good to feel good!

The changes I have made have been worth it and are long-term lifestyle changes.

"The best project you'll ever work on is you!"

UNKNOWN

Your life depends on it.

There is no going back now!

*"ANTs" is a term coined by Dr. Amen and stands for anxious, negative thoughts

Part I

Defining the issue of inflammation and autoimmune

Chapter 1

What is a health coach and why did I become one?

(I am Cheryl M Health Muse)

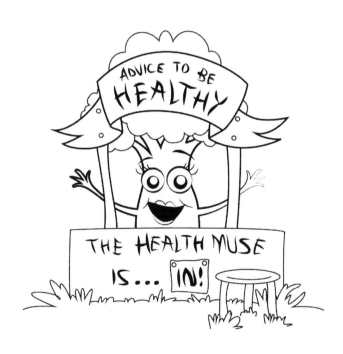

Dousing the flame of inflammation:

THE BIG TAKEAWAYS ON "WHAT IS A HEALTH COACH?"

- This book proposes a complete change in lifestyle to heal your inflammation and protect the health of your family.
- I have made these changes in my health, and I am almost free of pain.
- This approach can be overwhelming and a bit daunting at times. A Health Coach can keep you on track, inspire you to make the change, encourage you along the way, help you over the obstacles, and lead you to sustainable wellness.
- Health coaching is a relatively new field, but one that is quickly finding its place in the health care field as a way to help people reverse the damage from disease and find wellness again. Coaches can spend time with you to inspire the long-term lifestyle changes that your doctor doesn't have time to discuss.
- A health coach practices "compassionate" care. They will take the time to listen and "hear" you, encourage you to dig deep into yourself for your own answers, and guide you to make lifestyle changes that will change your health.
- I am committed to helping others find wellness again. We don't have to live on pills or live with pain. We can come out the other side of inflammation to a healthy, happy and full life.
- I know that "it feels good to feel good again," and I want to inspire you to feel good again too!

So, then … what is a Health Coach, or in my case A Health Muse, *smile*?

From Wikipedia

> "**Health coaching**, also referred to as wellness coaching, is a process that facilitates healthy, sustainable behavior change by challenging a client to develop their inner wisdom, identify their values, and transform their goals into action. **Health coaching** draws on principles of positive psychology and appreciative inquiry, as well the practices of motivational interviewing and goal setting."

Health coaching is a relatively new field, but one that is quickly finding its place in the health care field as a way to help people learn more about wellness and also to assist in reversing disease and to find wellness again. Coaches can spend time with you to create lifestyle changes that your doctor doesn't have the time to discuss in depth. This is also, probably, not your doctor's area of expertise. (Doctors typically receive only ½ a day on Nutrition in Medical School)

A health coach is a member of your health team that fills the gap between what your doctor has discovered and what you need to do to implement the changes needed to improve your health. A health coach can also be a guide to continued wellness incorporating new elements – all the things you need to do to replenish your soul, your life balance, ANTs[13], breathing, stress, organic eating, removal of toxins, sleep and, cooking etc.

Your health coach can help inspire and guide you to do the things you control for your own health. As an example, if I were your health coach, I would guide you to clean up your gut, which is the gateway to health; then work with you to clean up your world, and start to purge the toxins from your life. I would guide you to eat "real" food, organic if possible, and cook simple, nutritious meals to give your body beautiful fuel to heal. I would educate you on labels, food choices, lifestyle, stress, ANTs*[14], improving your sleep, and any number of other topics where you need help to improve your wellness. I would encourage you along the way to make sustainable changes. And we would discuss all of the avenues for you to explore to find joy in your life again.

If you are reading this book because you have inflammation and pain, a health coach can guide you back to feeling great again. A health coach can help you make changes so that autoimmune issues are not expanding and multiplying.

A health coach practices "compassionate" care. They give you attention; they listen to you; they acknowledge that you know your own body better than anyone; they will encourage you to dig deep into yourself for your own solutions and guide you to make lifestyle changes that will lead you back to wellness.

Working with a health coach would help prevent you from getting additional diseases from inflammation because it would help you heal the core issues. It would stop the progression of the diseases you do have, and turn you around towards health.

I have two autoimmune diseases, Type II diabetes, and undefined autoimmune disease. Once you have one autoimmune disease, apparently, it is not unusual to get another. If left untended, autoimmune diseases become increasingly violent disruptors to your health.

The information in this book is the result of 5 years of research, and I hunted and pecked all over the internet to find it. I was motivated; I refused to spend the rest of my life in pain.

Gaining this knowledge was an integral part of my healing, but it wasn't easy to find all of this information. I saw a need to gather all of this into one place. I wanted to share what I have learned in one book.

I listened to every symposium offered by the Functional community, on Diabetes, Thyroid disease, healing leaky gut, the adrenals, on detoxing for a healthy liver, on the importance of sleep, on gluten, on detoxing heavy metals and on fat and weight loss. I also was treated and learned from two Chiropractic doctors with degrees in nutrition and certification in functional medicine, from a certified Health Coach, and from a Functional MD. As of this writing, December 2016, I feel 80% better. If you do the things outlined in this book, you should start to get well.

Once I started to feel much better, I decided to go back to school so that I could help others with similar issues. I am committed to helping others. I decided to become a Health Muse (Coach). I took the HCTP course at **The Institute for Integrative Nutrition**® to get certification and a more formalized approach to health. I believe that they are best in the country for Health Coaching skills.

My new education along with my research did not create my wellness. It led me to where I needed to go and gave me a beginning understanding of what I needed to do. I knew I needed a team to help me along my path.

In my opinion, you will need a functional practitioner to run the tests you need and give you in-depth medical advice. My body has a lot of idiosyncrasies that my doctor has discovered with cutting edge testing, and literally, she has saved my life.

Once you know what is occurring in your body, as your coach, I could help you sort it out, and be a team member with you and your doctor.

My new knowledge allowed me to partner with my healthcare professionals and we were all important parts of what I needed to do to heal.

The health professionals noted in Part 6, Chapter 29, were all essential to my healing. Following them is part of my journey.

The body is complicated. I am a bit like an onion. For each layer where we find malfunctions in my body when the next layer is peeled off, there is something new to address. I am working with my Functional Doctor at this moment to chelate heavy toxic metals, as well as pesticides and herbicides, (I am loaded with them) and next up we will attack mold in my body. I learn more about my body every day.

If you are going to a conventional practitioner, this book will teach and help you own your own health. More than ever, you will need to be involved in your health. This book will allow you to encourage your doctor to implement things that will help your progress. You will be entering uncharted territory in some cases with your doctor, and you will need to be knowledgeable so that you can help your doctor delve deeper into the causes of your disease. A health coach could serve as an intermediary.

So, if you read this book, why would you still need me as your health coach?

Let's say; you need to make a trip to Slaplovia (a fictional location). You need to do business on your trip that will be integral to your success. You buy a guidebook to read on the plane on your way there. But still, you go alone. You didn't know the language or the pitfalls of traveling in this country, and even with a guidebook, it is a bit daunting to explore alone. You don't want to take wrong turns and end up somewhere that you don't belong. You have many questions along the way, and no one to ask. You don't even always know what you are looking at as you are working towards achieving your goal.

I want to be your tour guide to make your journey as enjoyable as possible, and to help you avoid "tourist traps" or in this case "pitfalls" along the way. Unlike a tour guide, you have hired me. I am not getting kick-back from the merchants, I recommend.

My role as your health coach will be especially helpful since I have lived through this process. I have been through everything in this book, so I understand at ground level how to help you. I have already jumped over most of the major hurdles that you will face. I have learned much of the language, and I know the route.

To get started, you will fill out an in-depth health history, and we will spend 1+ hour going over the keys to your health. This hour is *free* and kind of like a first date. You need to see if you can work with me, and I need to be sure that I think I can coach you. This hour is entirely devoted to listening to you. I will ask a lot of questions and act like an investigative reporter, to get the what, when, where, how, why and who of your health. Our first hour is not for advice; I will take lots of notes, and encourage you to share (and spill the beans). It is the time where I will listen to you and set a non-judgmental stage for us to begin our work.

If you decide to book the guided health care tour with me, prepare to roll up your sleeves and with my guidance, do the hard work. You will get as much out of our work together, as you put into it. You and you alone, are accountable for your life, and your own health. You will do the things that resonate with you that I suggest. You will develop your own strategies with my help. Everything is customized by you. You will set new **intentions** each time you meet with me, and I will hold you accountable to achieve them. My job is to lead you on your journey, point out the points of interest, give you background information, and answer questions. I will keep you focused so that you get as much as possible out of your adventure.

Each meeting will be a delicious hour all about you and your progress. It will be an hour that you will feel great about and feel proud of your accomplishments. It will be an hour where you get to show off what you have achieved. It will set your path for success one step at a time. We will meet every two weeks for one hour, either in my office or via skype or facetime or phone, to reset the course.

Expect to have "excuse-proof" accountability:

Each time we meet, you will review the **intentions** you agreed upon for the last two weeks, and update me on your successes and your challenges. We will brainstorm on where you have been and where you are going. I will make a few suggestions, to steer the bus, and you will commit to a few new **intentions** for the next two weeks. You will communicate what you want to learn on your tour, and I will be right beside you to help you implement these goals into the program. You will make progress one step at a time, and hopefully enjoy every moment of it. And we will do it with humor and joy.

We will celebrate your successes together.

I will listen to and "hear" what you are telling me so that together we will find solutions that you can maintain that will solve your health problems. I will direct you back to your health care professionals (your doctor, nutritionist, functional practitioner, whoever is on your team) when we need their expertise.

As your health coach, I will teach you to "own" your health, and become your own health advocate, no matter who these other health professionals are. I will join YOUR team to help you implement healthy habits. We will incorporate the advice from your doctor into our work together.

You have pain; that is why you bought this book, and you want to feel great again. Are you ready to implement the changes you need to do in order get well again?

You would not hire me to be your Health Muse because of my BA from Berkeley, or even for my health coaching credentials; you would not hire me for all of my management and coaching work experience. Now mind you, it doesn't hurt that I am "The self-proclaimed subject expert" and that I wrote this book. My life experiences will certainly help me ask you the right questions to guide you to where you want to go. You should hire me because I have lived through everything that I want to encourage you to do, and I can help you find your path to health. I will be a great tour guide, and your tour will be customized to you.

Even with all of the information in this book, you probably have not figured out how to do it all on your own, to cross the finish line. You are bound to have lots of questions. This book is the self-guided tour, but most of this information is foreign to you, and you will need guidance to make your wellness adventure all that it can be. You will hire me to get real results and to avoid taking wrong turns. I am suggesting changes that you can do and that your doctor will encourage, that will get results.

"Sometimes the smallest step in the right direction ends up being the biggest step of your life. Tip toe if you must, but take the step."

SIMPLE REMINDERS[15]

So, are you ready for change? Are you ready for transformation? You have to believe that you have the power to change your life if you could just see that path. I am here to be your Muse and help you find it.

I have been where you are, and am closer to who I want to be than ever before. Allow me to help you create that for yourself.

There is a lot here to sort through. I am committed to helping you regain wellness, and I can hold your hand and keep you accountable so that you reach your health goals.

"Circumstances in your life that hold you back are simply patterns that no longer work. Change the pattern, change your life."

MASTIN KIPP **DAILY LOVE16**

Remember,

"It Feels Good to Feel Good,"

and you CAN feel good again.

Chapter 2

You can't change what you don't understand - Inflammation

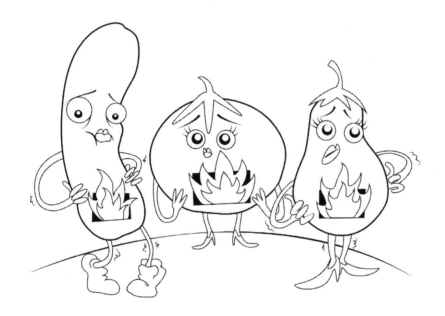

Dousing the flame of inflammation:

THE BIG TAKEAWAYS ON INFLAMMATION

- Identifying what your pain is and what to do about it.
- Identifying the shift in paradigm and how to find wellness specialists that can help you.
- Identifying and getting past your "already always[18TM]"
- Becoming your own "Who said of the greatest magnitude[19]."
- If necessary, finding a Functional MD who will treat your inflammation by healing your gut. Educating you on new approaches if you are working with a conventional MD.

Let's talk about inflammation and then autoimmune disease.

Soon after I hung up my "The Health Muse Is In" sign, *smile*, I started meeting a variety of people suffering from inflammation, but they didn't recognize that's what it was.

I understand this. I didn't recognize my health issues as inflammation or as Autoimmune. I had an inkling, but my conventional MD gave it no credence.

A couple of the people I have met, seem to be on the brink of going from inflammation to Autoimmune, and one had an autoimmune disease, Rheumatoid Arthritis, full bore.

People are resigned that as they age, they are going to feel a lot of pain. They seem to think that pain is their lot in life.

When and if they do decide to do something about it, the decision is to go to the doctor (of the conventional type) and get pills.

Their MD, in the current model of health care, is "The Who Said of the Greatest Magnitude." In our culture, doctors are all knowing. The current model isn't questioned. The way things have always been done is the way most Americans want to proceed. They don't even consider that there could be a better way. It's not in their vision of their "known truths."

One friend is actually on seven different pharmaceuticals, and still feels lousy and still has the pain. In addition, now, she is also having a reaction to one of the pills; she has a rash from head to toe.

These people are all part of the majority of Americans who do not seek a different way. This is what they know. They want to continue to take the pills and they pray that one of them will be the "magic" pill. The pills do offer some relief but come with horrible side effects. These people live in hope, and they have never considered anything else.

I have also met three different Moms with children suffering from acute sensitivities. They are cooking separately for these kids. The rest of the family is still eating the SAD (the Standard American Diet), and the sick child is rebelling and eating "normal" food whenever they can away from home. They want to be like everyone else even though it makes them sick, really sick. These children have conditions that are worsening, and the mothers are frustrated and don't know how to proceed.

None of these people wanted to hear that if they changed their diet, and took a sensitivity test, so they knew what foods to avoid, a big portion of their battle would be won. They didn't want to change. They saw it as deprivation. They would rather see a conventional doctor and take a conventional approach of taking pills, even though they recognized that they are still feeling lousy. It is the way things are done.

In the case of the sick child, the mother isolated her child, and it never occurred to her that the entire family could eat a clean, healthy menu with the sick child, so that the entire family would be healthier. With family solidarity, the sick child would gain strength from his family, and his wellness would begin. The healthy children would remain healthy and the sick child is included.

The chapter on autoimmune disease (Part 1, Chapter 4) will teach you what the disease is, and how it happens in the body. But you need to be open to new ways to look at your pain, food, your doctor, and your health.

"At any moment you have the power to say: "this is not how the story is going to end"

CHRISTINE MASON MIL[20]

So, first we have to figure out if you have inflammation. I was oblivious. Some of these things were obvious, but I didn't realize this was inflammation, nor did I know what to do about it.

So, let's start with this:

- Do you hurt?
- Do you have joint pain or stiffness?
- Do you have muscle pain?
- Are you getting headaches?
- When you look in the mirror, are you having good days and bad days? You look like yourself on good days, and on bad days you are swollen and puffy?
- Do you have brain fog, especially when you get up in the morning? Does it take a cup of coffee or two or three to get your brain up to snuff?
- Are you suffering from swelling, especially around your ankles? (I can also feel it in my hands and fingers and see it on my face.)
- Are you often constipated?
- Are you bloating, belching or passing gas?
- Are you tired when you get up?
- Do you have asthma?

Do you have:

- Water retention, skin puffiness
- Digestion issues
- Itchy ears or eyes
- Throat tickle, irritation or coughing
- Stuffy nose, sinus trouble, excessive mucus
- Acne, cysts, hives or rashes
- Ruddy, inflamed-looking skin
- Eczema or Psoriasis

These are all signs of inflammation. They are not to be ignored. Whatever form they are showing themselves into the outer world, they are doing damage in the inner world of your body as well. If you suffer any of the symptoms above, then it's time to make changes.

You have three choices:

1. Ignore all of the signs, and just go with the pain.

2. Go to a conventional doctor and get pharmaceuticals that mute the pain, but often do not cure it.

3. Embrace the new paradigm that real food can heal your body and that if you change your lifestyle, you can thrive. With this choice, preferably you find a Functional MD to locate the "root cause." You also find a health coach that can guide you along your new path. (See my chapter on what a Health Coach (Part 1, Chapter 1) is and what a Functional MD is (Part 1, Chapter 3).)

Remember the old adage, the definition of insanity is to do things over and over again the same way, and expect a different result.

I believe there is really no choice. The only acceptable way forward is #3.

Now I am sure that there are some excellent conventional MD's who will want to dig deeper, instead of just prescribing pills. Unfortunately, pills are usually the main tool in their tool box.

So, how do you do this?

It starts with getting you past your "already always ™."

Interesting phrase.

Some years ago, I had a business partner who had been through **Landmark Forum**[21]. It was human potential training, somewhat like **EST**; she thought it was a bit abusive but that it inspired change. It was NOT my thing. But she had a couple of phrases that she used from her training that I really loved, and one was to get past your "already always." Landmark used a term in their program that was similar for "already always thinking™".

So, what did my friend mean by "already always?" We think we are open-minded, but the reality is everything we hear and everything we believe, is filtered through previous experience and through what we have been told about ourselves. We now reinforce that in our minds. "Already always" is our "known truth," about ourselves and about the world, even if it is totally false. Unless we can break through that and look at the world through new eyes, nothing changes, we go back to our "already always." Before we can begin, the blinders must come off.

As a start, don't listen to everything your mind tells you. It is not the truth. It's just some idle chatter to keep you in your "already always." It tears you down, so that you stay in your "known truth," which has become your comfort zone.

"Don't believe everything you think."

ALLAN LOKOS, *POCKET PEACE: EFFECTIVE PRACTICES FOR ENLIGHTENED LIVING*[22]

Next commit to finding a new way to change your perception. You need to open your eyes, see the world from a new point of view, and change your filters. Changing your perception is practically impossible to do on your own. As a Health Muse, I can help you do this, but let's give it some thought right now, on lots of ways to approach this, for the purpose of this book.

See how many of these concepts you believe already, and then we will go from there:

- You don't want the pain anymore.
- Real food gives the body nutrients.
- You need to eat more real food and less junk food
- You know you should avoid fast food.
- You have an inkling that processed food is not good for you.
- You know that sugar is bad for you.
- You realize that Conventional doctors only spend an average of 5-12 minutes with you
- Generally, at the end of hearing your complaint, the doctor prescribes a medication. There is little lifestyle information given.

- You are frustrated when you leave the doctor's office. You remember symptoms you forgot to mention to him.
- You believe that each pharmaceutical has risks and downsides. Just listen to the drug advertising on TV, you know, that list of ailments that the announcer says real fast with small print on your screen and with very pleasant visuals. Advertisers know most people watch but do not listen to commercials. They aren't joking. All of those things can and do happen to people who take their pills.

If these things are all things you know on a gut level, then, what would it take to change your "already always." *What do you have to lose to change?*

Try this for only for a month and see how you feel? Could you commit to eliminating junk food, eliminating processed food, staying away from fast food, eating organic as much as possible, cooking, sitting around the table with your family at dinner eating healthy, eating local produce whenever possible, eating all of the colors of the rainbow, and eliminating sugar, just for one month?

This book is shining a light on the things you can do to reclaim your health yourself. Without pills.

To be clear, I am not suggesting that you stop taking any medication that your doctor has prescribed. But I am suggesting that you view food as health care, and medicine as sickness care and you start to change. Change your thinking, change your approach, and change your body.

Be informed. Be a participant with your doctor in your health. Whether your doctor is Conventional or Functional, be aware of what can you can do, so that you feel good again.

I think if you try these things for one month, you are well on your way, because you will feel so much better.

Implementing what is in this book, will be too much to try all together, but for one month could you follow my food recommendations? It's the fastest way to convince you that food is Medicine and that food can heal your pain.

Now some of you will want to take the plunge and do it all at once. I was sick and tired of feeling sick and tired, so I jumped in with both feet. I was motivated.

But I needed help and an accountability coach to teach me what to do and coach me along the way. I hired a health coach.

It was such a great experience; I went back to school. I am now a certified health coach so that I can guide and inspire you to make the giant leaps towards health that I made.

Others might want to do this in baby steps. Then you need a coach to keep you on track until the results become obvious and the lifestyle change is permanent.

You can move at your own speed. It gets easier as you gain momentum and start to feel good again.

What I suggest you do as you read this book is take a yellow highlighter pen and highlight the easiest things that you could implement right away. It took me 5 years to make these changes, and I am still changing things out to less toxic things that I discover along the way.

Take baby steps, but begin today.

When the first steps are accomplished, take a different colored pen and go through the book again and highlight what you will commit to purge next.

One step at a time.

Try it; you'll like it. *smile* Your body will vote YES.

The key is to do enough of the steps that you can "FEEL" the difference. Feeling better is the key that will give you the momentum to get well.

This isn't about some new "diet." This is about the necessity of making a lifelong lifestyle change. We will discuss how to do this and still have a yummy life. But, once you start to feel better, there is no desire to go back.

We are going to talk about discovering what foods you are sensitive to, and eliminating them. And we are going to discuss all of the toxins that you are surrounded by in your life, and I will help you clean them out, category by category. Only then will your body have the opportunity to thrive again.

You need to become your own "Who Said of the Greatest Magnitude." **You**. Not your doctor. You need to own your own health, and you need to "listen" to your body. It's a complete shift in mindset.

This doesn't mean that you won't form a partnership with your doctor. You need them. But it is a partnership. You become an active participant. You own your own health.

Start with food. Food can heal you. Or it can kill you. Your choice. You decide.

And then we will go from there.

Chapter 3

What is the Functional Medicine Approach?

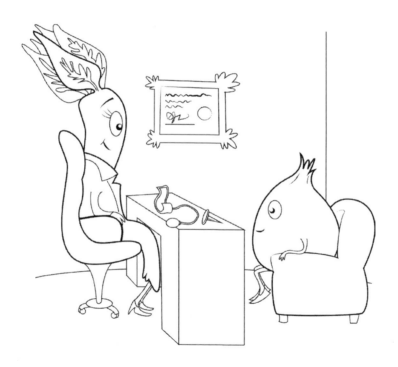

Dousing the flame of inflammation:

THE BIG TAKEAWAYS ON FUNCTIONAL MEDICINE

- Conventional medicine is broken when it comes to inflammation and autoimmune disease. Conventional doctors did not learn to include nutrition and real food in their bag of tricks in medical school.
- Healing inflammation begins in the gut.
- Instead of fitting your ailments into a round hole that pops out a pill, a functional doctor "looks for the tack"[24] – the root cause of the medical issue.
- Functional MD's are fully accredited physicians. They have had additional training and accreditation in "Functional" medicine.
- They might still prescribe Pharmaceuticals, but drugs are only one tool in their toolbox.
- They don't wait for you to be in a completely diseased state to take action. In other words, if your cortisol is low, but not at disease level (Addison's) they still look into what the root cause of the hormone deficiency is, and seek to heal it, before it reaches the diseased state.
- Functional doctors view the body in total; they don't focus in on one specialty system. They want to heal the whole body at the root.
- They believe that Food is Medicine.
- They are innovative and creative with the possible options available to regain health.
- My functional MD saved my life.

What is the Functional Medicine approach? Reflections on my own journey to health

I am often questioned about my enthusiasm for Functional Medicine. There is not a widespread awareness yet of this new branch of medicine.

To put it bluntly, this new approach to medicine saved my life, so it's worth me explaining.

Functional Medicine has been the cornerstone to my journey to wellness.

What lead me in the functional approach direction?

I was sick, and everything in my body hurt. I tried to research and give myself a diagnosis, and although I thought it was autoimmune related, I didn't seem to have all of the symptoms of any of the well-known branded diseases. It wasn't MS, or Lupus, or Fibromyalgia. It wasn't Rheumatoid Arthritis.

When I talked to my conventional doctor about it, at first she thought it was in my head, but to humor me, I was sent to the leading expert in autoimmune diseases at USC. He kind of snickered ... and offered me steroids. He pointed out that I didn't have all of the symptoms of any of the known autoimmune diseases, and when I turned down the steroids, wanted me to take Aleve twice a day.

It wasn't that my conventional MD didn't want to help me. She had simply been taught to examine the symptoms and prescribe a pill.

Ok, so the pain got worse. I discovered I had diabetes and was given pills for that. And my hands started shaking, so I saw experts for that. I was diagnosed with Essential Tremor. No drug, no cure.

As I mentioned in my opening chapter, I went to a DC (Doctor of Chiropractic) who had his degree in Nutrition. He made a significant change to my diet, and some of the pain subsided, but many symptoms continued. I couldn't lose weight. He finally told me I was very sick and he didn't know how to help me.

This ended up being a gift. I decided to do my own research and be in charge of my own health.

I watched the first Autoimmune Summit four years ago by Dr. Amy Myers, a conventional doctor who had been trained in Functional Medicine. Almost all of the presenters had been sick and had gone on their own journey to find something other than their initial training in conventional medicine, so that they could heal themselves. They found Functional Medicine, got certified and became Functional doctors. This new training gave them an entirely different approach. Each presentation seemed to conclude that it all started in the gut.

The gut? Could my road to health really be as simple as healing my gut?

So, I found my own Functional Doctor. She was trained conventionally. She too wanted a different approach to help her patients find wellness. She too had gotten sick and was looking for a better way.

It ends up it was not as simple as just healing my gut, but it was absolutely the place to start. This was a giant leap for me towards wellness.

This is what I have learned along the way.

Conventional Medicine is broken when it comes to inflammation and autoimmune disease.

As a nation, we have one of the worst infant mortality rates, one of the worst rates of diabetes, one of the worst rates of obesity; for the first time in history, our lifespan is decreasing, allergies, autism, chronic disease, inflammatory diseases are all on the rise at frightening rates. As a country, we are 28th in life expectancy but spend twice the amount for health care than any other country.

The old paradigm of seeing a doctor, getting a diagnosis, and then taking pills, not only does not treat the disease, but usually offers little relief and often causes additional problems.

Functional doctors are conventionally trained and they have gotten additional training in a new approach, the functional approach. They can still offer conventional approaches because of their initial training, but Functional Medicine is root cause medicine. A Functional doctor doesn't just want to identify the symptoms, give it a name and then a pill. They want to find the dysfunction and then find the "root cause" of the dysfunction, and they generally start with the gut. This is the definition from the Institute of Functional Medicine website.[25]

- "Functional Medicine offers a powerful new operating system and clinical model for assessment, treatment, and prevention of chronic disease to replace the outdated and ineffective acute-care models carried forward from the 20th century.
- "Functional Medicine incorporates the latest in genetic science, systems biology, and understanding of how environmental and lifestyle factors influence the emergence and progression of disease."

This doesn't mean that they avoid using conventional pharmaceuticals, but drugs are only one tool in their toolbox.

As Susan Blum MD explained in her book on Autoimmune disease[26], if you are sitting on a tack, a conventional doctor says wow, you are sitting on a tack, and gives you a pill that camouflages the tack and brings some comfort. But the tack remains. And sometimes the pill causes additional problems down the line.

A Functional Doctor becomes an investigator to find where the tack is and remove it. The first step in the process is to heal the gut.

It ends up I do have an autoimmune disease. There are at least 100 of them, many with names I never heard of and many more without names at all yet. In my case, I caught it early, so it didn't become full blown autoimmune. And we didn't need to give it a name to find a treatment. Mine was called undefined autoimmune disease. I also have Type II Diabetes, which unbeknownst to me, is also an autoimmune disease. Once you get one, it is not unusual to get others, if you don't heal the root cause.

A Functional Doctor starts to heal the body with real food, and with real nutrients and then looks to have the patient find balance for the body.

By healing the gut, finding the food and drug sensitivities and toxins that are destroying the gut and then removing them, and by rebuilding healthy bacteria in the gut, sometimes the whole battle is won. In my case, I got immediate pain reduction, but still had problems, so my Functional Doctor started investigating further to find the other tacks that were destroying my health.

"There is no magic pill, but there is lifestyle change that reverses chronic disease."

ANDREW SAUL FROM THE **FOOD MATTERS** FILM

If you are willing to make lifestyle changes, you can regain your health. Changing how I ate and lived has been extremely rewarding.

One thing for certain, healing my gut was the key to healing 70% of my pain. Healing the gut involves:

1. Feeding your body real live food, preferably organic, so that there are no herbicides or insecticides going into your gut destroying your good gut bacteria.

2. Eating all of the colors of the rainbow for their different nutrients.

3. Eating clean meat (grass fed, grass finished, and hormone, steroid and antibiotic free). (Ethically raised; for many reasons, least of all to end the obscene suffering the animals are put through. And, you don't want the animal's stress hormones.)

4. Eating local as much as possible, to get the most nutrients available from a freshly picked item.

5. Testing for and eliminating food sensitivities. This was a biggie for me. I have a long list of irritants and removing them created instant relief. Even today, if I accidentally eat something on my sensitivity list, I can blow up overnight, gain 5 pounds in 12 hours, and the pain returns to my muscles and bones. I get brain fog. My ankles swell. My face gets puffy. They are obviously a big part of my issue.

6. Rebuilding the lining of the gut (review the chapter on autoimmunity, Part 1, Chapter 4).

Ends up, the body is resilient, if given proper nutrients to help it heal, it can start to heal itself. All of the toxins need to be removed. We need to eat organic. All of the chemicals that are going into our processed and fast foods need to be avoided. Real live food is the biggest key to healing and sustained health. **Food Is Medicine**.

Other differences Conventional VS Functional

- My conventional doctor tested for allergies. The test was a strip down my back. The only thing I was allergic to was the adhesive tape that held the allergens. Allergies are things like an allergy to peanuts, or to shellfish. The reaction is immediate and can be life threatening.
- My functional doctor tested for sensitivities. Bingo. I had a huge slew of sensitivities. Now we had a place to start to heal my gut.
  Sensitivities are reactions to foods or chemicals that happen more slowly and subside slowly. They impact the gut lining (leaky gut) and can create an

autoimmune reaction in the body. Sensitivities still do damage to the body, but they are usually not immediately life threatening. They are what starts the process of inflammation, and what causes the immune system to go wild and start to attack your own body.

Allergies and sensitivities have different inflammation markers, and sensitivity tests are looking for these various markers.

- My cortisol levels were low. Since I wasn't at "disease" level, Addison's disease, then there was nothing to do, according to my conventional MD. My Functional MD ran a test for my DHEA level, which was completely depleted (DHEA is what the body uses to create new Cortisol), she added a DHEA spray to my daily routine, increased my selenium, also good for my thyroid, had me work on my stress with exercise and breathing. The result: My cortisol is now creeping back into a healthier range.

- My health history made my functional MD question my level of toxic metals in my body. We tested. I was loaded with lead, mercury, copper, cadmium, arsenic, and more. Before we attempted to detox the heavy metals we looked at my ability to Methylate. From testing, we discovered I have two genetic anomalies to methylation, so knowing that my body doesn't detox easily, we worked on improving the methylation process; we detoxed my liver, increased my vitamin B-12, had me remove my amalgam fillings at a biological dentist, did vitamin intravenous treatments (called a Meyers cocktail) for several months (with vitamin C, Magnesium, B Vitamins, Folate, and more) and now we are detoxing the metals out of my body.
My conventional doctor never noticed or questioned the fact that I can't detox, or that I had a methylation issue or that I was loaded with toxic metals. Having the MTHFR anomaly to my DNA is cutting edge medicine. Even when it is written up in specialty journals, it can take 17 years before the trickle-down effect allows the research to be seen by a conventional doctor.

- I ran the **23 and Me** genetic test. Most people do it to find genealogy; we did it for DNA information. Knowing that you have weirdness's in your DNA doesn't mean that you are going to get all that stuff. It does, however, raise markers to be aware of. So, the first new thing that was obvious is that I still have high elevated estrogen in my body even though I am well into menopause. My methylation anomalies were also blatant on the DNA markers.

My journey continues, and I am sure that we will make other fascinating discoveries about my body as I follow my path. Without my Functional MD, I would still be miserable in my body, my health would be deteriorating, and I would have little or no hope.

Instead, now, I want to help others make lifestyle changes that will help them either avoid disease, and increase their wellness over the course of their lives.

My blood pressure has come under control, but my diabetes and weight are still challenging. I do understand now, though, that until my entire body works in tandem, it will be difficult to fix these issues. One system at a time, we are moving towards solutions.

One other aside, my Functional MD has a specialist in her office that is a miracle worker and does Frequency Specific Micro current on the body, which has reduced my pain dramatically. This specialist is also functionally accredited, a chiropractor, nutritionally trained, and she has been instrumental in my healing.

"Magic happens when you don't give up, even though you want to. The universe always falls in love with a stubborn heart."

JIM STORM

You need to be diligent to find solutions, and you need an open mind to find answers. Think outside the nine dots.

Functional Medicine literally saved my life. ("Yes, Susan, there is a Santa Claus.")[27]

Side note: How to find a functional doctor[28]:

Go to the Institute of Functional Medicine website, find the practitioner tab, and put in your zip code. **Voila!**

Chapter 4

What is Autoimmune Disease?

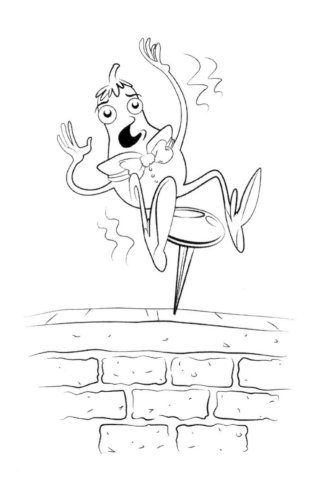

According to medicine.net:[30]

> **"Autoimmune disease:** An illness that occurs when the body tissues are attacked by its own immune system. The immune system is a complex organization within the body that is normally designed to "seek and destroy" invaders of the body, including infectious agents. Patients with autoimmune diseases frequently have unusual antibodies circulating in their blood that target their own body tissues.

Dousing the flame of inflammation:

THE BIG TAKEAWAYS ON AUTOIMMUNE DISEASE

- There are over 100 different diseases under the autoimmune umbrella.
- The disease is rising rapidly in the US, and Conventional Medicine is failing to stop the epidemic. It is now the 3rd leading cause of death in the US. Women have 75% of the disease.
- There has been a shift in lifestyle, our food, our environment, and our lives that have created the conditions for this disease to flourish.
- Healing the disease starts with the gut. You can get better.[31] You can reverse the disease or lower the volume on your genetic expression.[32]
- Defining "leaky gut" and what to do about it
- We need to purge the toxins out of our lives if we want to heal a leaky gut. Our food, our cosmetics, our cleaning supplies, our water, our over the counter drugs, our minds, our toxic sleep and even possibly our relationships have toxins that need to be eliminated.
- There are proactive things that you can do to reset your path to wellness.

Autoimmune diseases are the number one health malady in the United States. In total, there are more than 100 of them. They are the #1 cause of body dysfunction in our country.

WHAT ARE THEY?

- Autoimmune Addison's disease
- Chronic Fatigue Syndrome Immune Deficiency Syndrome (CFIDS)
- Crohn's Disease

- Degos Disease
- Dermatomyositis
- Dermatomyositis – Juvenile
- Discoid Lupus
- Fibromyalgia – Fibromyositis
- Grave's Disease
- Guillain-Barre
- Hashimoto's Thyroiditis
- Insulin Dependent Diabetes (Type I)
- Juvenile Arthritis
- Lupus
- Meniere's Disease
- Mixed Connective Tissue Disease
- Multiple Sclerosis
- Psoriasis
- Raynaud's Phenomenon
- Rheumatic Fever
- Rheumatoid Arthritis
- Scleroderma
- Sjogren's Syndrome
- Ulcerative Colitis

And many others with long names I don't understand.

Autoimmune also includes symptoms that don't fit into a named peg hole yet. I was diagnosed with an undefined autoimmune disease.

Newly added to the list:

- Diabetes Type II (just one of my autoimmune issues)
- Alzheimer's
- Some skin conditions
- Cardio Vascular
- Possibly even autism
- Parkinson's

And more to come.

Cancer is just being explored as a possible leaky gut issue.

Autoimmune Disease is rapidly on the rise in the US. It is estimated that 50-75 million Americans have it; 75% of them are women. Women are 3 times more likely to get the disease than men.[33]

There has been a 300% increase of autoimmune disease over the last 50 years. There are now 250 million with the disease worldwide. Autoimmune is the 3rd leading cause of death.[34]

What is causing it? What can we do about it? Why is the conventional medical community failing to stop this epidemic?

The traditional approach of naming the syndrome and giving the patients pills is not healing the body. It is not putting the disease into remission. It is covering up the symptoms, and it is often exasperating the problem.

Conventional medicine approaches the disease as a problem with specific body system. Whatever forms of autoimmune their patient is dealing with needs a specialist in that area. They believe that it is all genetics, and they believe that it cannot be reversed.[35] Conventional doctors treat autoimmune disease with harsh medications that turn the immune system off. We need our immune system, so that can harm the body.

Drugs are causing new problems in the body; this was something that I understood. Both of my parents had unusual diseases that eventually killed them, and the drugs prescribed made their conditions worse, not better. In my father's case, the pharmaceuticals became a bigger issue than the disease.

A Functional MD *wants* to find what is triggering the immune system to over-react, and then turn that off, the trigger, not the entire immune system. **They look at the body as a whole.**

In the last couple of decades, there has been a shift in lifestyle, in our food, and in our environment. They are all having a diverse effect on the human body.

The Functional Medicine approach to Autoimmunity is to bring balance back to the body. Not to name the dysfunction, necessarily, but to enable the body to heal itself wherever there is inflammation.

The key is to heal an inflamed gut. A functional MD doesn't just treat the complaint; they want to heal what is causing the complaint. (Remove the tack)[36]

There are more bacteria in the gut than there are cells in the body. These bacteria send messages to all functions of the body. There is even a brain-gut connection. The gut is your second brain. (And I just read that the brain is your second gut. Fascinating.)

SO, WHAT IN THE WORLD IS LEAKY GUT?

My sources of information are Dr. Tom O' Bryan DC, CCN, DACBN,[37] Dr. Susan Blum, MD[38], and Dr. Amy Myers[39]: all leading functional experts on Autoimmune Disease and then of course from my own Functional team and my own experience.

60-80% of our immune system is in the gut. The gut has a semi-permeable lining wall that is only one cell thick. On that wall are little tiny fingers, like a shag carpet. Over the shag carpet is something like cheese cloth.[40]

The bacteria in the gut break our food down into amino acids. A healthy gut lining, allows friendly amino acids to go into our system as particles that are recognized by our immune system as friendly particles.

Your immune system is set up to identify "name tags" according to Dr. Susan Blum. All your cells have name tags so that your immune system knows that they are supposed to be there, so it doesn't attack them.

If our digestion isn't working properly, if we don't have enough "good" bacteria, large chunks of food are in the gut, not yet broken down into amino acids.

Leaky gut is where the link in the chain of your gut breaks, and tiny little holes allow these larger food particles to pass through the wall and into your bloodstream. These holes remain open, allowing the larger food particles to pass through. These holes need to be healed and closed for the disease to stop progressing.

Digestion is supposed to destroy the "name tags" on food. But if the food isn't broken down properly, and if it is left in big chunks, it can cause holes in the cheesecloth barrier over the shags and get into the blood system. These particles enter your bloodstream" and your immune system can't identify them and goes "whoa", sees them as the enemy, and attacks.

Over time, you can build up antibodies against any food that is slipping through, chicken, tomatoes or a long list of other foods that are your sensitivities, so your immune system perceives more and more particles as the enemy.

These particles do a form of molecular mimicry. Our immune system sees them as foreign invaders similar to other cells in the body. These particles could look like thyroid tissue, or other tissues in the body, and our immune system then attacks not only the "foreign" invader, (the larger food particle that is slipping through) but also the tissue that is being mimicked. Our immune system starts to attack our own body.

The immune system is signaled to attack different body systems, wherever our greatest vulnerability is and where the tissues being mimicked are. For me, it was my muscles, my liver, and my pancreas. For someone else, it might be their thyroid. It is what causes MS and Lupus, and it is what causes Rheumatoid Arthritis and diabetes. It causes brain fog and eventually it causes Alzheimer's. It is now thought to be what causes Parkinson's. It might even cause autism. It causes healthy body functions to break down.

WHAT CAUSES THE LINK TO BREAK AND THE GUT WALL TO BE PUNCTURED?

1. Genetic vulnerability – A conventional MD sees this as the only cause. The reality is that it is only one of the causes.
   If you don't eat real live green food, the light switch can be turned on.
   These are the markers you genetically inherited, but they don't need to be turned on unless your body functions are not working properly.

2. Environmental triggers
   There are several possibilities.

   - Food sensitivities – Common foods that create sensitivities are corn, soy, dairy, gluten, grains, legumes, eggs and nightshades.

- Toxins (they have invaded our lives and are everywhere. Read further in this book)
- Chemical (there are 80,000 chemicals in our environment. There are 1700 more chemicals introduced into our environment every year.[41] The safety of the chemical is left up to the manufacturer. The process for approval takes less than 3 weeks. There are 126 toxic chemicals in personal care products alone. 25% of women use 15 daily. On average, a person uses 9 of these a day. The company doesn't have to prove that it is safe, and these chemicals are actually shown to be very harmful in studies done by The Environmental Working Group (EWG)
- Wheat, whether you are tolerant of gluten or not, we are not born with an enzyme to properly digest wheat ... and over time it can cause permeability in the gut wall. Studies are just coming in that this could also be the result of glyphosate (the stuff Monsanto is spraying all over conventional and GMO crops and feeding to us)
- It could be smoke in the air from local fires.

1. Sugar, alcohol, caffeine, GMOs, Roundup© (by Monsanto) are all believed to contribute to leaky gut

2. Toxic metals

3. Radiation

4. Stress

5. Some drugs, steroids, antacid, NSAIDS, acid blockers, are all believed to contribute to leaky gut[42]

6. Infections, parasites, candida

The problems begin when the body burden from all of these toxic factors become too great for the body to handle.

Your gut heals itself every seven days, but eventually it can't keep up. Gut bacteria can change in as little as 48 hours, both positively and negatively.[43]

WHAT ARE THE EARLY SYMPTOMS OF LEAKY GUT?[44]

- Poor digestion
- Pooping too loose or too hard, or back and forth.
- Fatigue
- Depression
- Food Sensitivities
- Headaches
- Bad skin
- Pain, especially joint pain. I also had muscle pain.
- Swelling, for me it was most noticeable around my ankles, my fingers, and my face.

WHAT YOU CAN DO TO HELP YOUR BODY AND HEAL A LEAKY GUT

1. Get a food sensitivity test done, and whatever they are for you, avoid all of them like the plague. It is possible, after your gut heals for a while, that you can bring them back into your diet one at a time but for now, they are gone, you can't eat them. You could also do a Food Elimination test, eliminating all of the usual suspects (dairy, grain, nightshades, soy,) and then reintroduce them one at a time six months later and observe your body's response.

2. Food can be the slowest form of poison if your body has become sensitive to it.

3. Eliminate toxins in your life. We are going to discuss this in depth in the next part of my book.

4. Get tested for infections in your gut.

5. In my opinion, avoid GMO foods. Avoid as much conventionally grown food as possible. It can't be good for the body to eat herbicides, pesticides or

fungicides. If those things are killing bacteria and bugs on our crops; they could also be killing the good bacteria in our gut.

6. Eliminate sugar. It is more addictive than cocaine and heroin. It is what causes triglycerides in your body. It is destroying your liver and your pancreas. It is doing damage to your brain and your kidneys. It takes 2-4 weeks (my experience) (one sugar expert says two months) to detox off of sugar, and then you don't care about sugar at all. Sugar also increases appetite and turns off your body's ability to know it is full, causing it to crave more sugar.

According to Dr. Susan Blum:

- "Sugar triggers your immune system. This is a stressor that can eventually damage the way your immune system functions, which then leads to an autoimmune reaction."[45]
- This includes high glycemic foods like soft drinks, juices, foods made with white flour and processed sugar, candy, cookies, ice cream, etc.
- There are good and bad gut bacteria. One of the things that need to be increased is the good gut bacteria. You will need a good probiotic and also a good prebiotic. Probiotics add the good guys to your lower intestine. Prebiotics feed the good bacteria.
- For probiotics, you can eat plain yogurt and kefir. You can also eat fermented foods and drink Kombucha. Raw sauerkraut and miso soup are also good probiotic foods.
- For prebiotics, you can eat foods like jicama, onions, garlic, leeks, rye, chicory, blueberries, raspberries, plantains, bananas, asparagus, dandelion greens and artichokes.

There are also good prebiotics and probiotic supplements to take. I take Klare. I also take Klare enzymes so that I maximize the good nutrients going through the gut wall.

Other Dr. Susan Blum Suggestions:

FOODS THAT HELP HEAL THE GUT

- "Healthy fats, including ghee and coconut oil as well as olive oil, avocado oil. The only healthy fats that are specifically gut healing are ghee (contains the SCFA butyrate) and coconut oil (anti-candida), and for anti-inflammatory action, the omega's EPA/DHA/GLA, olive oil."[46]
- Glutamine: A good source comes from pastured animal protein, such as beef and chicken.
- Organic Bone broth from grass fed cows or pastured chickens and turkeys
- Glutamine is also in beans, cabbage (raw), beets, spinach (raw), and parsley,
- There are high quality supplements available to boost your availability of Glutamine which allows the liver to replenish its supply in 60 days. After 60 days, eating the correct foods noted above, should allow the body to make its own.

Dr. O'Bryan says that if you stop throwing gasoline on the fire, the lining of the gut begins to heal.[47]

From personal experience, eliminating food sensitivities, eating live green food, eliminating toxins, and eliminating sugar, gave me relief in as little as 2-4 weeks. No pills, I just gave my body the tools it needed to heal itself. AMAZING!

This was not my total solution, but it certainly put a big dent in all of the inflammation I was suffering within my body. My functional doctor keeps peeling the layers of the onion of my health. We have discovered toxic metals; we have discovered additional biome issues; my body doesn't detox properly; I am not absorbing nutrients properly. I have a fatty liver. I am a work in progress. But I am well on my road to recovering my health.

"I regret eating Healthy today," said no one ever.

UNKNOWN

ISN'T THE BODY AMAZING?

When you heal your gut, and give your body beautiful nutrients so that it can function properly, the pain starts to subside, the fire of inflammation goes out, and you are on your way to wellness once again.

For more information, I strongly advise watching the Dr. Tom O'Bryan's film *"Betrayed"* about autoimmune disease and how the current model of medicine is failing to stop the autoimmune epidemic. This documentary is invaluable to someone struggling with autoimmune disease and inflammation. You need this information to help you get well. I bought it for future reference.

There are often Autoimmune symposiums given on line by the leading experts in the functional approach to the disease. Get on the mailing lists of the doctors listed in Part 6, Chapter 28, and you will be notified when they are happening. Much of what is discussed in these free lectures are cutting edge. This was where I started my journey before I knew any of the information in this book.

There are 3 excellent books on Autoimmune Disease written by my references above. Dr. O' Bryan and Dr. Blum and Dr. Myers that were invaluable to me to understand the nature of my ailments and what to do about them.

The Immune System Recovery Plan: A Doctor's 4 – Step Program to Treat Autoimmune Disease Dr. Susan Blum, MD Scribner; 1 edition (April 2, 2013)

The Autoimmune Fix Dr. Tom O'Bryan Rodale Books; 1 edition (September 20, 2016)

The Autoimmune Solution: Prevent and Reverse the Full Spectrum of Inflammatory Symptoms and Diseases Dr. Amy Myers, MD Harper One; 1 edition (January 27, 2015)

I was lucky and found an amazing functional team in Los Angeles; my doctor Shilpa Sayana, MD and Susan Spizer, LAC. Their office now also has a functional practitioner working with children. They are in Studio City, California. They are looking to hire additional Functional practitioners.

Functional doctors are in high demand. If you are unable to find one to help you reverse your autoimmunity, both Dr. Susan Blum and Dr. Amy Myers have remote programs with backup staff that can lead you through the most important initial steps. I put contact information in Part 6, Chapter 28, Amazing people leading the way.

Don't get discouraged. You can change your lifestyle and how you eat and begin to reverse the inflammation that is causing your disease. You can positively impact your health.

Chapter 5

One last thought Flares

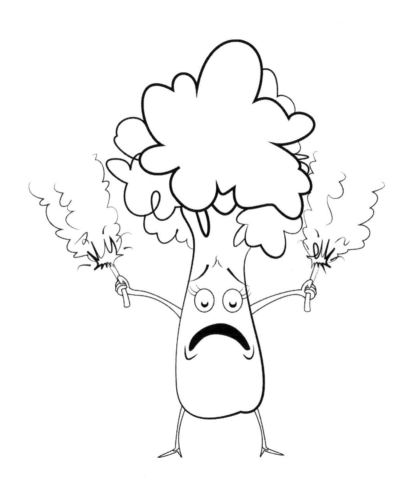

Dousing the flame of inflammation:

THE BIG TAKEAWAYS ON FLARES[49]

- Flares will happen, and for a short period you will have pain and inflammation again.
- You may or may not know what caused it.
- After reading this book, you will understand how to move through them.

Even if you do the entire protocol outlined in this book, this is not the end of the story. For me, it cured 75% of my pain. And trust me, eating this way and cleaning out the toxins has been totally worth it.

There is no doubt; it feels good to feel good.

But as my functional MD and I pull each layer off the onion, there is something else underneath that needs attention. I had not paid attention to my body for a very long time.

Once you clean up your food and clean out the toxins, if you are still not up to snuff, you will need a Functional MD to help you uncover the rest of the mysteries of your body and find all of the tacks.

I am still having difficulty losing weight, so we are working on my liver, methylation, my thyroid, and my estrogen. I now understand that the entire body must work together, organ by organ, system by system, for the weight to resolve itself. (I strongly recommend Dr. Libby Weaver's book *Accidentally Overweight – The 9 elements that will help you solve your weight puzzle*. Hay House, Inc.; 1 edition (March 1, 2016) The book is greater than the title suggests. Dr. Libby explains how each organ system needs to heal and how they all need to work together for optimal wellness. And when wellness is achieved, weight loss occurs.)

And one other note, I do want you to celebrate when you start to feel good, even great.

But beware, suddenly you can eat something that you didn't know was on your sensitivity list and have a "*flare*." Or you try a food on your list and still react to it. Or there is a forest fire in the area, and your body reacts to the smoke. Or you are in a stressful situation, and suddenly you gain 5 pounds overnight and have inflammation and pain again.

Flares don't last long, and now you fall back on everything you have learned in this book. In a few days, you are back to feeling great again.

I immediately increase my intake of Curcumin BP, Quercetin, and Resveratrol, all anti-inflammatory substances, to douse the flame of new inflammation.

It's probably nothing that you did wrong. Your body just catches fire more easily than people who have never dealt with inflammation. Be kind to yourself. Go back to basics, and wellness will return once again.

In some ways, I think flares keep me grateful that I have come a long way and I am not going back. All of this work to get well and living a healthier lifestyle plus eating real food is worth it.

A flare just creates a new set of hurdles to understand and jump over, but there is no doubt, you now know you can get over the hurdle. And "it feels good to feel good."

Part 2

Toxins

Cleaning up the toxins in your life.

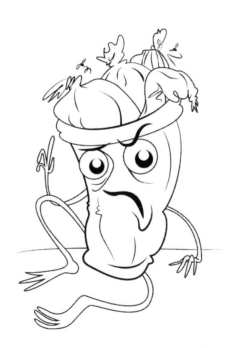

Dousing the flame of inflammation:

THE BIG TAKEAWAYS ON
INTRODUCTION TO TOXINS

- Big business — Big Agriculture, Big Pharma, and Big Food are all loading our world with chemicals that are poisoning us, and our government is not protecting us.
- Many of these chemicals are blocked from use in the European Union.
- These toxic chemicals are responsible for the fact that we rank 37th[51] in the world for health.
- People with knowledge who speak out are demonized.
- Often our media is not covering the story. There is too much money in advertising to buck.
- Too much money is changing hands at every level.
- You need to become your own advocate and get informed to protect your own health and body.
- You need to become an "army of one"[52] Join me.

Toxins. Probably the biggest surprise, when I started on my get-well journey, was discovering that there were so many toxins in everything I ate and used in my life. It has been rather disheartening to find that we are being poisoned and that our Congress and Food and Drug Administration are allowing it to happen.

Big Chemical, Big Food, and Big Pharma have billions of dollars to protect. They do their own studies that are manipulated to show that they are making healthy foods and using innocuous chemicals. These self-serving studies are accepted by our government as fact. These products are destroying the environment. They are killing the bees, which are critical to our crops. They are marketing falsehoods like GMOs are feeding the world. They are causing disease. They are destroying the soil microbiome. And they are making money hand over fist.

They are protected all the way along their path. Things that are not studied are given "generally thought to be safe" status. Synthetic chemicals are in our processed foods that give the body no nutrition, and often cause us harm, but taste good and often are purposely addictive. These synthetics are a less expensive route for big food to take. But as a result of the toxic fake ingredients, our bodies are starving, and disease is growing.

Conventional Doctors are often wined and dined by Big Pharma to educate them on pushing more pills. These pills have huge downsides and often are worse than the original disease. (Some of these medications do help, but pills are not the only solution.) No one has taught conventional doctors that food is medicine, and that toxins kill. Conventional doctors certainly mean their patients no harm, but they function under their own "already always"; it's how they were taught, and it's the only approach they know.

You have to take control of your own life and the lives of your families. Otherwise, we are just going to get sicker and sicker as a nation.

When choosing a path that resonates with you, be careful of Nay Sayers who declare that there is an absence of evidence to support your approach. Since Big Chemical, Big Food, and Big Pharma do their own biased studies, there might be an absence of evidence in following a real food approach, but what there actually is, is evidence of absence[53] …. Studies that are double controlled placebo double blind studies are rarely done on healthy options that have no money or profit tied up in their success. You won't find a study on the benefits of leafy green vegetables but your body will jump for joy when you feed it real nutrients, and that's what's important.

These are all my opinions after studying the situation for the last five years, to improve my own health. It is upsetting.

I will admit that I don't know that the independent studies that are contrary to the self-run studies Big Corporations are doing in their own interest, are scientifically sounder than the ones Big Corp is funding. I am not a scientist. But I tend to believe the independent scientific community over the self-serving studies that are being accepted. And, by eliminating these toxic substances from my life and my diet, my health has turned around. That is my proof and will be yours as well, if you take my suggestions.

Big business is out there demonizing the people who are taking a stand against them. They don't want you to know the truth. It would not be good for business. They are willing to destroy our lives and our environment for the almighty buck and will do anything so that you can't learn the truth. Some of the brave people that are taking a stand against them are targeted by the phony news (propaganda).

These heroes are often highly educated PhDs and advocates that are opposing big business.

People like Dr. Mark Hyman MD, who is one of the fathers of Functional Medicine; he is the Director the **Cleveland Clinic Center for Functional Medicine**. He is also the founder and medical director of **The Ultra Wellness Center**, chairman of the board of the **Institute for Functional Medicine**. He is a medical editor of **The Huffington Post** and is a regular medical contributor on many television shows including **CBS This Morning, Today Show, Good Morning America, CNN, and The View, Katie, and The Dr. Oz Show**. He has inspired thousands of people to wellness. He has written countless books, and he communicated all of the latest research. When I looked him up on Wikipedia, I was appalled. Wikipedia is sourced by whoever *wants* to write. They don't understand the Movement that Dr. Hyman is a part of at all. He is educating and helping millions of Americans. He was demonized. Shame on them.

I have seen them demonize countless others, like Del Bigtree, who took on vaccinations with his film **VAXXED**. My husband is a statistician. When we saw the movie, he was appalled at the lack of ethics in how the statistics were manipulated by the CDC for the drug companies. Del Bigtree was blocked from showing his film to a large audience. The media did not support him; they supported the CDC and big drug. They have demonized him. You should see the film and make your own decision. **http://vaxxedthemovie.com/** the movie is utterly frightening, and it is showcasing something hurting a significant percentage of our children.

There is also the doctor from Argentina who spoke out at The Hague Tribunal in the World Court, in Oct 2016 and found his office locked up, and his staff fired when he returned home. Big Money is impacting whistleblowers all over the world.[54]

There are countless others.

I fully expect that they will demonize me.

I am not a scientist. My BA is in English from Berkeley. My career was in retail and then designing jewelry for my own company. I am a subject matter expert only because of all of the research that I have done to improve my own health and the certification that I just received from The Institute of Integrative Nutrition®. My proof is in my health. I have gone from lots of pain to feeling good again.

Eliminating toxins has improved my life dramatically. So, I offer up these chapters as a guide. I write them as a way to introduce you to the dangers lurking in your everyday life. I do believe that it can improve your life if you also eliminate these things from your world. I have decided that I am not going to go deeply into what the chemicals are, but instead I will first explain the issue by category and then to offer suggestions to clean up the toxic waste in your life. Finally, I want to give you resources so that you can study it further. You need to take control of your life and do your own research if you are so interested. New information comes out daily. You need to stay current. You need to own what you can do to create a healthy environment, for you and your families.

There is nothing in this book that you could not find on your own by researching online. But this information is scattered all over the place. It has taken me five years to find all of this and to go through the trial and error of finding what works for me. I wanted to give you a place to start with all of the information that I have found by locating it all in one spot.

My greatest hope is that you try my suggestions and let your body vote. My bet is as you eliminate all these toxins from your world, your body will vote with me, and you will start to feel good again.

I do know that the only way that any of this will change is bottoms up with our dollars. If we stop buying these toxic products, big food, big chemical and big pharma will have no choice but to change. The change has begun. When both the House and the Senate passed the Dark Act, I realized that it had to be a grass roots effort or that it will never change. (*The Dark Act* doesn't want us to have easy access to know what GMOs are in our food. Although there is a complicated way now to know, it's pretty hidden from the general public, and difficult to use.) The Senator that sponsored the bill received more money for his campaign from Big Chemical than any other legislator. Big money talks, but it doesn't have to talk to us. We have our own minds and can fight back.

Howard Lyman[55], an ex-rancher, an advocate against what is happening with our meat, the inhumane way the animals are treated, the hormones and steroids and antibiotics that the animals are given ,and the disgusting food they are raised on, made a statement that each of us need to become an "army of one"[56] if we plan to change the system. He states:

"Remember there are no rules for living on our planet, only consequences, and Nature Does Not negotiates."

HOWARD LYMAN[57]

There is a lot of information here to digest. You are not going to accomplish all of this overnight. It took me five years to make the changes I am suggesting, and I was highly motivated. I wanted to get well. And I am not done. I keep finding new categories of toxins in my life that need to be examined.

I am also learning that I must revisit the latest information every year. I am learning a great deal writing this book. Manufacturers change formulas, and new testing is performed regularly.

The faster you clean out the toxins and dump them from your life, the better off your life, your body and your family will be. My suggestions may be perfect for you, or not. If not, go back to the resources I am suggesting. It is not about following my lead. It is about you finding what works for you. There are many options. Whether or not this works for you depends on "your individual mind and body, and your preferences, and your stage of life."[58] In other words, you are unique, so what works for me may not work for you. But do start to purge the chemicals and the toxins. And at the same time be kind to you. Take baby steps if you need to, but systematically, throw these things out. When your health improves, you will truly have a great deal to be grateful for and to celebrate.

I am joining the war. I am an army of one. We all deserve better. Come join me.

Ready? Then let's start with food.

Order the dumpster; there are toxins to purge

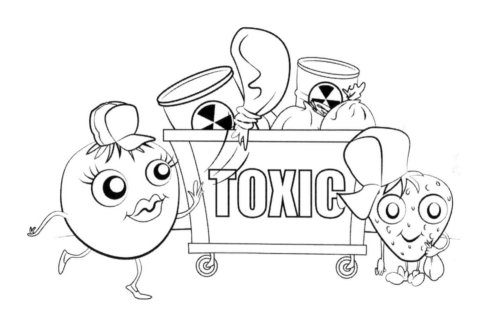

"Our greatest vulnerability lies in the amount of misinformation and misconditioning of humanity. I've found the education systems are full of it."

R. BUCKMINSTER FULLER[60]

Dousing the flame of inflammation:

THE BIG TAKEAWAYS ON PURGING THE TOXINS FROM YOUR LIFE

- You are living in a toxic dump in all areas of your life. Your food, your cosmetics, your cleaning supplies, your water, your drugs, your mind, your sleep patterns, sometimes even your relationships are toxic and killing you. They are all creating inflammation and disease,
- Food is medicine. Our conventional approach is disease care.[61] There are times when conventional medicine is needed and works well. But for inflammation and autoimmune disease much of our healthcare system is broken.
- You need to become responsible for your own health and become informed for the sake of your health, the health of your family and the sake of the planet. You need to be proactive to take back your health.
- The paradigm has shifted. Just as you know that the world is not flat, in your gut, (a play on words, but true) you know that conventional medicine, when it comes to inflammation and autoimmune diseases is not curing us anymore. There is no magic pill.
- Diets don't work. There is no quick fix. We have to start eating real food again.
- You must cook. It is not an option. We need to know what we are putting into our mouths. Cooking is the only way to control what goes into your food. We also need the community of sitting around the dinner table together.

If I told you, you were living in a toxic dump in all aspects of your life, what would you say? Would you want to clean it up?

Are you sick? Is a family member sick? Even if you are healthy, with no signs of pending sickness, this book is for you.

I am here to shake up everything you know about food, calories in calories out, eating fat, doctors, pharmaceuticals, weight loss and health, your cosmetics, your personal care products, your shampoos, your cleaning products, your everyday essentials. Your beliefs about food, health, conventional doctors, medicine and your favorite products are all outdated.

That's a big statement. But it's true. And there is now science to back it up. These are my opinions:

- Gone are the days where doctors are curing all illness with drugs. Many drugs give some temporary relief, but often cause side effects and other long-term issues.
- Gone are the days where you need to try every diet on the NY Times Best Seller list to lose weight. These approaches haven't worked before, and you already know they won't work now. There is a better way.
- Gone are the days of calorie counting.
- Gone are the days of beating yourself up for not losing weight.
- The days of being addicted to sugar, corn syrup, fructose, and the blue, pink and yellow packets of chemical sweeteners should be gone forever. Sugar is even more addictive than cocaine, and sugar lights up the same part of the brain that cocaine and heroin do.
- The days of stopping for fast food on the way home from work should be gone forever. There is absolutely no food value in most fast food, but there is a cocktail of very unhealthy chemicals.
- The days of avoiding good fats like butter, olive oil, coconut oil, lard, tallow, avocado oil, grapeseed oil and ghee should be gone forever. They are good for you and essential to how your body and your brain function.
- The days of using corn oil, vegetable oil, *Crisco*, canola oil, safflower oil, and soy oil should be gone forever (including canola-olive oil mixtures) (and they need to go into the dumpster.) We switched to these oils as a result of a massive marketing campaign back in the 50's and 60's. It was false marketing.
- The days of buying junk food and processed food to fuel your body should be gone forever. Again, little or no food value, but tons of toxic chemicals. Nothing in these foods gives your body any nutrients to function. Eating these foods is starving your body.

- The days of eating food with ingredients that you can't pronounce should be gone forever. Those ingredients you cannot pronounce have no food value and are all chemicals that your body can not use. They are often toxic.
- The days of believing government and industry telling us that GMOs are feeding the world should be gone. It is simply false. They are making you sick. No matter how they justify it, conventionally sprayed produce and GMO's are foods that are getting you to consume pesticides, herbicides, fungicides and toxins. These toxins kill the bugs in our outside world, and they kill the good bugs in your gut. They are also killing our bees. They are destroying our soil microbiome and reducing needed minerals for life.
- The days of eating conventional animal meat from inhumanely raised animals, filled with hormones, steroids and antibiotics should be gone forever. This includes most factory farmed fish, and even chicken eggs that are not fully pasture-raised. And when you eat this meat, all of the animal's stress hormones go into your body, in addition to lots of nasty toxins.
- The days of getting antibiotics for the flu, (a virus, so it does no good) for colds, for other ailments at the drop of a pin should be gone. They have their place and their purpose but need to be used more judiciously. They kill the bad but also the good bacteria in your body. And if you take them for every hiccup, they aren't effective when you need them. With all of the antibiotics used in our food sources, we are reaching a crisis where the antibiotics are not working anyway.
- The days of using over the counter drugs indiscriminately should be gone forever. The harm they are doing to your body is simply not worth the relief they provide. Some are difficult on the liver; others are difficult on the stomach and the gut. There are other natural ways that work with your body, and I will address these later in this book. I have created my own non-toxic medicine cabinet.
- The days of buying name brand cosmetics and thinking they are good for your skin should be gone forever. They are also not making you beautiful. Cosmetics are not regulated for toxins and are used on the largest organ of the body, your skin, so the toxins are absorbed and dangerous. The usual detoxing organs like the liver and kidneys now have to deal with this added toxic burden.

- The days of using perfumes and colognes should be gone forever. Again, they are loaded with toxins.
- The days of buying that favorite shampoo and conditioner that was making your head itch should be gone forever.
- The days of buying most cleaning supplies at the grocery store or big box retailer should be gone forever. The most toxic thing in your home is your laundry detergent, but probably all of your cleaners are toxic.
- The days of buying anything with nasty chemicals in them, your food, your cleaning supplies, your personal care products, your cosmetics, should be gone forever. This includes toxins in some clothing, upholstery, and carpeting. This even includes toxins in our personal care items, like tampons, and Q-tips which are made from GMO cotton.
- The days of drinking water from the faucet should be behind you. Your water is probably loaded with toxic fluorides and toxic chlorine. In some communities, the water is loaded with lead. (And far more widespread than Flint, MI.) You need a good filter system. Check with your city or county what your local water report states.
- You even need to clean up toxic thoughts, your toxic relationships, and your toxic habits.
  - You need to work on your anxious mind, your worry, your *ANTs*[*62].
  - You need to change your toxic habits and get 7-8 hours of real sleep. Your body uses that time to do tune ups all over your body.
  - You need to quit smoking.
  - You need to stop drinking excessive alcohol.
  - I know marijuana is legal now in some places, but unless you are using it medicinally, the verdict is not in on how it affects the body, so limit your use.
  - You need to focus on all the things you need to do to replenish your soul: your life balance, *ANTs*[63], breathing, stress, movement, meditation, healthy relationships, healthy thoughts, spirituality, and joy, to have a healthy life.
  - You need to practice being grateful for your body and your environment, and in general for how blessed you are for your life.
  - You need to temper the toxic stress you are dealing with on a daily basis.

And why is this important to get reeducated about and then change?

We are a very sick nation, health care costs are through the roof, and if you get educated and change how you think and react to all of these areas and if you take control of your own food and environment and own your own health, you can save your family and maybe even help save the world.

In the United States:

- 10% of the population currently has diabetes.
- 33% of our population is pre-diabetic and will have diabetes in 5 years.
- 39% of our population has or will get cancer: 1 in 2 men and 1 in 3 women are expected to get cancer in their lifetime.
- 53 million Americans have an autoimmune disease, mostly females. (This includes 1 in 5 females and 1 in 7 males.) And it is growing at ever increasing rates, to the amazement of the health community.
- 160 Million Americans are overweight or obese
- New childhood diseases are rapidly escalating, including Juvenile Diabetes (Type I Diabetes), Type II Diabetes, Fatty Liver, Autism, Allergies and Sensitivities, ADHD, and more.
- I saw a statistic that it has been estimated that by 2025, 50% of our children will have some form of autism. Yikes!

We have to do something. You have to do something. This situation is simply unacceptable.

I have always hated generalizations. There are many conventional doctors that care and that truly want to make a difference. They have good intentions as they practice their trade. They are using every tool that they have in their tool box to help and care for their patients. They want to positively treat their patient and help them heal.

But often, the tools they have in their tool box are pharmaceuticals. This needs to change. There are other tools now that involve eliminating the toxins and eating real food.

I am also not saying all conventional doctors are uninformed, but many are. Current research is usually published in specialized journals, and it is estimated that it takes seventeen years for this research to reach non-specialized journals[64]. They are also stuck in their "already always."

I am not saying all pharmaceuticals are bad or useless. They have their place, and conventional medicine is important if an operation is needed, or something critical is going on, bones are broken, to fight infection or "to buy time to find the tack.[65]" (Explained in the chapter on autoimmune disease, Part 1, Chapter 4.)

A conventional specialist MD is important for gynecology or heart care or when there are physical things wrong with the body. They are important for organ malfunctions.

However, the entire premise of Conventional medicine needs to be reevaluated. Doctors are indoctrinated in a specific approach; their model of health thinks that the body is a machine. It assumes that one method always works and that they need to define the ailment and then prescribe the pill.

This approach is left over from the Industrial Revolution. In the early years of medicine in our country, Medical schools were built by Pharmaceutical companies that were funded by billionaires like Rockefeller[66], who had a vested interest in selling their drugs.

Doctors are not taught anything significant about nutrition. They get ½ of 1 day in medical school about food. They have not been taught that food is medicine.

"Medicine is not Health Care. Food Is Health Care. Medicine is Sick Care. It is time we see it for what it is"

UNKNOWN[67]

The human body is not a machine. It is time to accept that this model no longer serves all of our needs. It is not working.

What I am saying is it's time for you to take your own health into your own hands, and do some research about what you and your family are being exposed to. You deserve to know, and your family deserves to be healthy. Knowledge is power, and

I want to get you started on that path. I want to open your eyes. I want you to be responsible for your body and your health.

We vote with how and where we spend our money.

That's what this book is all about. I want to give you beginning tools to clean up the toxic waste in your life.

Big Food, Big Pharma, Big Chemical, the government, and your doctor should no longer be (what I call) the "*Who said of the greatest magnitude*." You know the ones with almighty knowledge that are after your "best interest" if you just listen to them. Doctors will tell you that they know they are not God. You alone can be the judge and monitor of what is in your best interest. Work together with your doctor, but study and be a contributor to your health.

This is a massive shift in a paradigm. And this will take a moment for you to get your head around; I am asking you to apply the principle that the world is not flat to the world of health and medicine.

"You never change things by fighting the existing reality. To change something, build a new model that makes the existing model obsolete."

R. BUCKMINSTER FULLER[68]

I want to participate in building a new model that makes the existing model obsolete.

1. The first step is to identify the problem.
2. The second step is to inspire you to make the change.
3. The third step is to teach you the tools for implementation.

This book is going to take a look at each of the toxic areas in your life that are not usually considered by conventional medicine, give you suggestions and teach you how to clean them up, and give you the tools to take control and ownership of your families lives. I will teach you to replace the toxins with products that are friendly to your body and our environment.

By the time we are finished, if you follow my suggestions, your toxic load should be well on its way to being empty. Let your body vote. Eliminating these toxins should allow you to start to heal.

These changes will not all occur overnight. It takes the time to purge all of these toxins out of your body, your home, your mind, and your life. As you run out of a product you have been using, replace it with a better choice. It will take some experimentation, and it will take a commitment to get well. You will learn to "read" your own body.

You don't want to be sick, and you aren't going to take it anymore!

I encourage you to do the best you can to eliminate as many toxins as possible one step at a time.

As you read this book, I suggest you have a yellow marker pen. Use it to highlight the things you can implement easily and start there. This is a process. You cannot do it all at once. But you can take little steps each week to create a healthier life for yourself.

Reread my opening chapter **"Dedication, How to use this book."** There are great suggestions given as to how to roll out incorporating this into your life.

"The path isn't a straight line; it's a spiral. You continually come back to things that you thought you understood and see deeper and deeper truths."

JOURNEY ON EARTH[69]

Acknowledge and celebrate each change that you make and be kind to you because change takes time. Do the best that you can do. Be vigilant (now I say it, *smile*)

Celebrate every change that makes your body sing. Each step you take today will bring you closer to a healthier life for you and your loved ones.

If you are having trouble implementing the suggestions in this book on your own, this is where I would come in as a Health Coach. There is a lot of work to clean all of the toxins out of your life, and as your coach, I can encourage you, keep you on the path, and hold you accountable to make the changes necessary to heal your inflammation.

Once you have cleaned up the toxins in your life, your doctor can help you clean out the toxins from your body.

As you work with me, we will find healthy solutions that are lifestyle related. Simple changes can make an enormous difference in your health. I am not a doctor, a nutritionist or a dietitian. As your certified health coach, I can help you in different ways from those health professionals. As your health coach, I will provide you the support to make the changes necessary for wellness. We won't just talk about food, and eating clean, and healthy recipes, we will talk about your food sensitivities, sleep, and all the things you need to do to replenish your soul, your life balance, *ANTs*[70], breathing, stress, and cleaning toxins out of your body, your environment, your cosmetics, and your life.

Working together, first, we will clean up your gut, which is the gateway to health. I will listen and "hear" what you are telling me so that together, we will find sustainable solutions to solve your health problems. We will spend delicious time together. **This is all about you.** I will teach you to "own" your own health, and you will become your own health advocate, to participate in your health with the other health professionals you have chosen for your team. I can also support you while you clean all of these toxins out of your life. (see my chapter on what is a health coach, Part 1, Chapter 1)

If you decide to work with me, prepare to roll up your sleeves and do the hard work. I will guide you to success. You will get as much out of our work together, as you put into it. You and you alone, are accountable for your own life, and your own health. You will do the things that I suggest that resonate with you. You will come up with your own strategies. You will customize this to you. I will help you find a pace for change that you can do and be proud of. You will set new intentions each time you meet with me.

None of this will interfere in any way with what your doctor is prescribing. These are changes that you can adopt for yourself.

With or without me, dump the toxins. Dump them as quickly as possible.

Once you reclaim your life, there is no turning back. Never forget how good it is, to feel good.

Getting well and feeling good are what this book is all about.

Part 3

Food

Chapter 6

Organic vs GMOs vs Conventional Farming

How do you choose what you buy and eat?

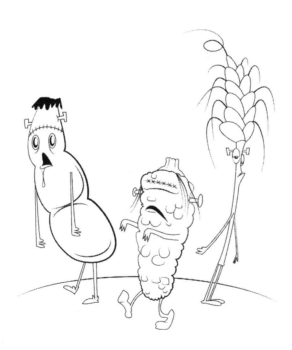

"If you don't take care of your body, where are you planning to live?"

DR. TONY GANEM, D.C.

Dousing the flame of inflammation:

THE BIG TAKEAWAYS ON ORGANIC VS GMOS

- The scientific evidence that is generally accepted insists that pesticides and GMOs are not harmful to animals or humans. These studies are self-funded by the chemical companies themselves.
- Brazil's National Council for Food and Nutrition Security just published a document citing 750 studies that show the environmental and health risks that are being ignored by countries regulatory agencies, in a lengthy report recently published in GM Watch, 2/27/2017 *The 750 studies that GMO regulatory bodies often ignore*. "Credibility damaging campaigns for researches and authors mentioning such hazards and uncertainties are also described."[72] "In the section on health risks, the book's authors note that the scientific literature shows "immune and allergic reactions" in animals and humans to Bt toxins of the type engineered into GM plants.[73]"
- It doesn't make sense to me that pesticides, herbicides, and bacterium grown inside our food could possibly be good for us, so my personal decision is to side with caution and avoid these foods.
- Food grown organically is closer to the way that Mother Nature intended. The human body operates as it is intended when we eat "clean."
- The question becomes, do you want to eat poison? Study or no study, could that possibly be good for you or for your families.
- Even a relatively small drop in market share for conventionally grown crops and GMO products will change the future of how our food is grown. Vote with your money. Vote with how you shop and with what you eat.
- Yes, organic food does cost more.

When this book is completed, my next project will be to pull together how to eat organic on a budget as an eBook. It is the #1 objection that I hear when I talk about eating organic. However, please consider, is there is a price attached to being healthy and disease free?

How much can you save in future medical bills? I save money by not eating out, not going to Starbucks, bringing my own food wherever I go, and cooking my own meals. And I save money by limiting my exposure to toxins. Eating organic has improved my health and cut down on visits to my doctor and the number of pharmaceuticals that I need to take on a daily basis.

I realize that I will not live forever. I do, however; want to have the best quality of life possible for as long as possible so that I can enjoy the ride.

To get started, I think we need to define terms:

"**Conventional farming**, also known as industrial agriculture, refers to methods of farming in which include the use of synthetic chemical fertilizers, pesticides, and herbicides and genetically modified organisms. **Conventional farming** is contrasted to **organic farming** as the latter responds to site-specific conditions by integrating cultural, biological, and mechanical practices that foster cycling of resources, promote ecological balance, and conserve biodiversity."

Organic farming is a form of agriculture that relies on sustainable techniques to enhance the natural fertility of a farm, including crop rotation, companion planting, biological pest control, and naturally-sourced fertilizers such as compost, manure, green manure, and bone meal."[74]

GMO definition from the World Health Organization

"Genetically modified (GM) foods are foods derived from organisms whose genetic material (DNA) has been modified in a way that does not occur naturally, e.g. through the introduction of a gene from a different organism. Currently, available GM foods stem mostly from plants, but in the future foods derived from GM microorganisms or GM, animals are likely to be introduced on the market. Most existing genetically modified crops have been developed to improve yield, through the introduction of resistance to plant diseases or increased tolerance to herbicides.

"In the future, genetic modification could be aimed at altering the nutrient content of food, reducing its allergenic potential, or improving the efficiency of food production systems. All GM foods should be assessed before being allowed on the market. FAO/WHO Codex guidelines exist for risk analysis of GM food."[75]

I chose to eat organic!

Whether or not to eat organic or to eat conventional produce (or GMO) is a very confusing decision. There is so much information available. It appears to me that much of what is available to read is "alternate news" i.e. "Fake News." As a regular human being, it's hard to sort through the facts and determine whether or not they are facts and make a decision as to what to buy and what to eat.

Since I am not a scientist and only a concerned citizen that got very sick with inflammation and autoimmune disease, I have made a cautionary decision to avoid as many chemicals as possible, in all aspects of my life. The good news is that taking this stance has reversed a great deal of my inflammation, and I feel great again. Eliminating toxins goes far beyond food, but food is a perfect place to start.

I am going to present the information that swayed me. There is no way for me to know if it is "real" news or not, but I want to give you the information that I have found that made me decide organic was the only way to go.

If you do your own research, you will find the things I am listing below, and you will find an alternate set of facts. Please do what you think is in your best interest. You own your health. Get informed.

I will admit I started with the point of view that eating pesticides, herbicides, fungicides or things that are modified which would never have occurred in nature, could not possibly be good for me. That was backed up by the information that I found. I present this information for your consideration.

These comments are my opinion. After doing my research, my decisions are as informed as possible.

There are so many toxins in our food; it's almost difficult to know where to begin. Every aspect of our food is contaminated, by different substances, for different reasons. It is my opinion after researching what is happening to our food, this is the biggest reason that our health is deteriorating. The United States is now 37th in wellness in the world because we are allowing toxins to enter all aspects of our food, as the European Union and other countries are banning these chemicals. We have also been invaded by toxins in many other areas of our lives. See Parts 3, 4, and 5 of this book.

Food is wellness. Clean up your food, and a big part of your inflammation battle is won.

So, let's start with how our food is grown. It's the best place to start.

Live Food, how it gives us wellness or makes us sick

Organic vs. Conventional

When I started my own journey to wellness, I was only vaguely informed on the difference between organically grown food and conventionally grown food. I also really didn't understand what GMOs were. Now that I have read everything I can put my hands on, I have no doubt that wellness begins with eating organic fruits and vegetables, preferably locally grown.

I will get into what I consider the horrors of GMO's (Genetically Modified foods) in a moment, but let's pause and discuss why organic is more expensive. This is the #1 objection I hear when people hear me say organic. Yes, it is a little more expensive to buy organic, over conventional (aka factory farmed) produce, but the long-term cost savings to you and your family in long-term health care costs could be well worth the price. You make your decision after you read this and do your research.

Why is organic food more expensive than conventional factory farmed food?

1. **No chemicals = more labor**[76]
   The Organic Farming Research Foundation explained it well: "The organic price tag more closely reflects the true cost of growing the food: substituting labor and intensive management for chemicals, the health and environmental costs of which are borne by society."

2. The rules of supply vs demand. There is a greater demand for organic than is currently available.

3. **Higher cost of fertilizer for organic crops**[77]
   "Sewage sludge and chemical fertilizers might not be something you want in your food, but conventional farmers use them because they don't cost much and are cheap to transport." (I find that disgusting.)

   Organic farming uses a more natural fertilizer that is more expensive to ship.

4. **Weeding by hand**[78]
   Organic farming does not use all of the chemicals that kill the weeds around their crops

5. **Crop rotation**[79]
   Organic farmers use age-old techniques of crop rotation. "Higher prices of organic cash crops compensate for low financial returns of rotational periods which are necessary to build soil fertility."[80] The benefits of crop rotation are healthier soils. Healthier soil produces healthier p*lants*. Chemicals are chelating the minerals we need from the soil and therefore also from the plant. Organic farming grows food that is richer in nutrients and minerals. (There are studies that show this is true, and there are studies that show this is false. It is logical to me that this is true, so in my opinion, this is a crucial technique).

6. **Longer growth cycle**[81]
   Organic produce often takes longer to grow, because they use no enhancers to speed up the process.

7. **Smaller volume makes farm to market more expensive**
   It also needs to be kept separate, which adds to the cost of transportation.

8. **Organic certification** [82]
   There is a fee to get USDA certified, and there are additional fees involved to comply with the USDA standards. It is more labor intensive to keep strict records that must be available for inspection at any time.[83]

9. **Cost of covering higher loss**
   There is expensive crop insurance. Since organic farming does not use synthetic pesticide, herbicides or fungicides, they are more susceptible to crop loss.

10. **Better living conditions for livestock**
    Organic livestock eats their natural diet, and organic farmers have higher

standards they need to comply with when the animal comes from organic farms. Organic feed is much more expensive than conventional feed.

11. **Organic food spoils more rapidly**
There are no chemicals in the food to slow down the natural process of spoiling. The life span is in tune with the way Mother Nature intended. This is a strong reason to buy organic as local as possible to ensure the plant is as fresh as possible.[84]

12. **Subsidies**
"Production-oriented government subsidies reduce the overall cost of crops. In 2008, mandatory spending on conventional farm subsidies were $7.5 billion while programs for organic and local foods only received $15 million, according to the House Appropriations Committee."[85]

My take-away from this:

- Food grown organically is closer to the way that Mother Nature intended
- Food grown organically is NOT using synthetic chemicals on the crops. It would be difficult for anyone to convince me that eating pesticides and herbicides could possibly be good for me. (More on this later)
- Organic food is ironically, more controlled by the US government than conventional farming. This is a good news, bad news scenario. It is good news that the government enforces organic regulations to protect me. The bad news is where the heck are they in protecting us from conventional food chemicals?

Since Big Chemical does their own biased studies, there is an absence of evidence in following an organic real food approach vs a conventionally produced vegetable or fruit. What there actually is, is evidence of absence – studies that are placebo controlled double blind studies are rarely done on healthy alternatives that have no money or profit in their success. You won't find a study on the benefits of kale, or spinach or bok choy or carrots, but your body will give you the evidence, and that's what's important.

In spite of some research that states there is no nutritional difference between organic and conventional produce, the studies do not touch upon the effect of the pesticides on the human body. Recent research in 2016 however does show a big difference in nutrients because organic food is grown in soil still rich in minerals.[86] [87] Soil that has been continually sprayed by herbicides and pesticides no longer has many minerals; the sprays chelate the minerals out of the soil.

If I understand it correctly, there were studies done that showed significant problems with pesticides and GMOs to animals and humans.[88] [89] The people who did those studies were fired, their careers destroyed, and their research was destroyed. Again, I have no way of knowing for sure is this is true, but it is certainly disturbing.

(It kind of smells like the Tobacco industry, doesn't it?)

So, where would you begin?

Start with buying organic produce using the **Dirty Dozen list+** and conventional produce from the *Clean 15* lists that are published by **EWG (Environmental Working Group)**. If the food is on the **Dirty Dozen+** list, and if the food is conventionally grown then it has a multitude of chemicals on it. If it is on the Clean 15, then it is relatively safe to eat from a conventional source.[90]

The EWG 2017 Dirty Dozen[91] plus (taken from 2015 data)

1. Strawberries
2. Spinach
3. Nectarines
4. Apples
5. Peaches
6. Pears
7. Cherries
8. Grapes
9. Celery
10. Tomatoes
11. Sweet Bell Peppers
12. Potatoes
13. Cucumbers
14. Cherry Tomatoes
15. Lettuce
16. Imported Snap Peas
17. Domestic Blueberries
18. Hot Peppers
19. Kale/Collard Greens

The EWG 2017 Clean 15

1. Sweet Corn
2. Avocados
3. Pineapples
4. Cabbage
5. Onions
6. Sweet Peas
7. Papayas
8. Asparagus
9. Mangoes
10. Eggplant
11. Honeydew Melon
12. Kiwi
13. Cantaloupe
14. Cauliflower
15. Grapefruit

These lists are a starting point for you to buy organic food. Stay updated, the lists change every year.

Once you read what I have to say about pesticides, herbicides and GMOs, I hope you will expand your list to include all of the fruits, vegetables, seeds, and nuts, fish, and meats that you consume, but you need to start somewhere, and this is the best place.

CONVENTIONAL FARMING

Conventional farming relies on synthetic pesticide, herbicides, and fungicides to increase the amount of the crop that gets to market. Use of these chemicals allows the crops to be bigger with less labor, which reduces the cost.

The pesticides being used have only been studied by the Chemical manufacturers for safety. Our government accepts these studies. Therefore, up until now, they have been "generally considered safe" by our Food and Drug Administration. Just a note, the people who have been at the head of the FDA for many years, are the past or future executives for **Monsanto**. Isn't that ducky?

In addition to the Dirty Dozen, the following foods are also heavily pesticide sprayed on conventional farms. I am noting which crops are GMO **Roundup Ready®** as well. I will get to **Roundup Ready®** (a trademark of Monsanto Company) further in this chapter, but for this moment in time, understand that GMO's have the insecticide or toxin bred right into the plant. (Not going to wash that off now, are you?)

- Wheat (gets drenched with Glyphosate to increase yield right before harvest, which stays on our wheat and goes right into the food it is intended for.)
- Canola *GMO* Roundup Ready° is a trademark of Monsanto Company.
- Sugar beets *GMO* Roundup Ready° is a trademark of Monsanto Company.
- Potatoes (have been tested with 35 different chemical residues on conventional potatoes)[92]
- Papaya
- Corn GMO Roundup Ready° is a trademark of Monsanto Company.
- Sweet Corn *GMO* Roundup Ready° is a trademark of Monsanto Company.
- soy (it's everywhere in processed food) GMO Roundup Ready° is a trademark of Monsanto Company.
- cottonseed oil *GMO* Roundup Ready° is a trademark of Monsanto Company.
- Zucchini
- Summer squash (There are 40 chemicals tested on a summer squash)[93]

This gets even more worrisome when you realize that the USDA scrubs and peels the vegetable or fruit before it is tested for chemicals.

I would buy organic, if at all possible, if the item is on the above list.

The chemical companies publish their own rigged studies[94]

I was asked recently if I was against science. Absolutely not. I am, however, against science that has been done for profit. Unfortunately we are dealing with science for profit in several areas of our lives now. This kind of science is being done by Big Chemical, Big Food and Big Pharma so we need to use our common sense.

Dr. Joseph Mercola, in his article *Healthful Foods You Should Never, Never Eat* October 4, 2011 states on his website, "Self-controlled studies by the chemical industry use various methods to create desired, but false or misleading, outcomes in scientific studies. Such tactics include using:

- "Inappropriate control groups.
- "The wrong statistical methods use incorrect detection methods.
- "Simply withholding negative results is another common tactic."

From what I have read, most of these studies have not been longer than 3 months. Yep, 3 months. There are no industry sponsored studies longer than 3 months to determine if there is a detriment to our animals or human health.

"Monsanto, one of the primary players in the field of genetically modified (GM) foods, wants you to simply trust them because they're 'experts' and their studies 'prove' their GM foods are safe. But these same experts also told you PCB's, Agent Orange, and DDT were safe, and we now know those claims were far from accurate."[95]

Again, these studies are being done by the chemical companies themselves and the government is accepting them as true. Good grief. How does that make sense?

The proof for me is also how sick the animals we eat have become. And the proof is in how sick we are becoming as a nation.

If you look at charts showing when chronic disease suddenly skyrocketed,[96] there is a direct correlation to when pesticides and **Roundup Ready**® (a trademark of Monsanto) GMO seeds were becoming a major player in the food supply. Now I explained to you earlier, correlation is not necessarily proof. The proof is that when animals are fed organic feed, they get well[97], and when we eat organic food, we do too.

What I can't determine is whether or not stressful animal practices are a confounding variable. The animals might be getting sick from a variety of circumstances. But to me, it is logical that insecticides and pesticides could certainly be a contributing factor. Remember, they are poison.

An interesting aside, I just read an article that states Monsanto serves organic food in their cafeterias in all of their facilities.[98] They do not feed conventionally grown food to their employees.[99] If this is true, do you want to be eating the pesticides that Monsanto doesn't want their employees to eat?

This is a quote right off **Monsanto's** own website. **"Is there a real difference?**[100]

"The only honest answer is: It depends. Clearly, if you specifically want your food to be grown without certain pesticides, technologies or additives, you may prefer 'organic' varieties."

I choose to prefer "organic" varieties.

There are dozens of different pesticides sprayed on our conventional crops. I just spent an hour trying to find a list of what they are, to no avail. I do know that one of them is Roundup© by Monsanto. But there are dozens of others, and often, in combination, they are more deadly than a single pesticide being sprayed on our produce.

Take a look at the warnings on the Monsanto Roundup© Label. I have put an endnote below so that you can find it easily.[101] Just pick up the bottle the next time you are in a store and read the label. Do you really want to ingest a poison that you need to be very careful not to touch or get on your skin or breathe, let alone eat it on your vegetables? I don't.

California has recently taken steps to require **Monsanto** to label *Roundup©* as carcinogenic.[102] A California court has given the go ahead. **Los Angeles Times** *"California gets closer to requiring cancer warning label on Roundup weed killer"* by the Associated Press 2/7/2017 "Monsanto had sued the nation's leading agricultural state, saying California officials illegally based their decision for carrying the warnings on findings by an international health organization based in France." That health organization is the **World Health Council.**

Some of these toxins remain in our environment and our bodies for decades. You will see an article quoted at the end of this chapter about what these chemicals are doing to our oceans, and how devastating that will be for our long-term survival.

These chemicals are infiltrating our ground water and our water systems, and are in our drinking water. Therefore, these chemicals are getting into our bodies through our food and our drinking water. And when these chemicals are sprayed on crops by crop dusters or other factory machinery, they are also polluting our air.

Just one of these toxins is **Roundup©. Roundup©** binds with minerals that we need for body function. Because of this, minerals are no longer available in the plant. The p*lants* are getting sick. We are eating nutrient deficient p*lants.* **Roundup©** makes the plant sick and weak, and since it binds with needed nutrients, it has the potential to make us sick and weak.[103] [104]

I have read that **Roundup©** interferes with detoxing by blocking enzymes in the body.[105] [106] This is particularly interesting to me since my functional MD has discovered I have a difficult time detoxing, so chemicals that are in my body don't have an easy pathway out. This is something that I am working on with my functional MD. We discovered that I am also not absorbing needed nutrients from my gut, so we have improved that by adding enzymes to my supplement regime. Now, this is all making sense to me.

According to Jeffry Smith, **Monsanto** knew all of this from their scientific studies, but they hid this information from the public.[107]

Monsanto also knows that **Glyphosate**, the key ingredient in **Roundup**© damages intestines in rats in as little as 10-15 days.[108]

As if this wasn't bad enough, **Glyphosate** is liberally used as a ripening agent on sugar cane and wheat. The plant is doused in **Glyphosate**, and then there is a greater yield, but all of those chemicals remain on the food and go into our food products (and eventually into our gut) in much greater amounts."

There was an ironic video[109] posted on Facebook some time ago, where a reporter asked a Monsanto scientist if **Roundup**© was safe. He stated, yes, it was safe enough to drink. So, the reported offered him a glass of **Roundup**©. The scientist declared "I am not stupid." The scientist turned red, stared at the glass for a moment, squirmed, started to sweat, and then got up and left. As he left, he called the reporter a complete jerk. Hmmm, if it's so safe why did he say he would be stupid to drink it? You decide.

Glyphosate has been named as a possible carcinogen by the **World Health Organization**. (And this information is what lead the **State of California** to decided that the label of *Roundup*© must have a warning on it, as reported above.)

There are additional toxins in **Roundup**© to make the Glyphosate more effective that are recently being studied and may have even more dire effects on the human body.

Are you beginning to understand why it is my opinion that it is critical to your health to eat organic? Even though there are few studies that prove me right, but when I think it through, there seems to be no way I will consider eating plants that have been liberally sprayed with pesticides and herbicides.

GMOS

So, let's discuss what GMOs are, and why it is possible that they are toxic to our bodies, our environment, our soil, our farm animals, our pets.

"If anybody ever tells you that we know with one hundred percent certainty that GMOs are totally safe to eat, they haven't done their research. There is no reason GM foods should be approved safe for consumption; we just don't know enough about them. We could easily feed the planet through organic, GMO free methods, there is absolutely no reason we need GM foods around."[110]

What is the nature of the toxins in GMOs?

GMOs are when the toxin is bred right into the plant. Yep, the plant is born with the toxin in its DNA.

How are you reacting as you read this? I was appalled. How could that possibly be good for us? My opinion.

Chris Kresser stated in a blog on his website **ARE GMOS SAFE?** November 30, 2012 "Are these chemicals harmful to animals or humans? It's impossible to tell at this point who has the right answer, and it's unnerving that there is so much controversy over the safety of a food product that is present in 60 to 70 percent of processed foods found in grocery stores."[111]

Jeffry Smith, the Founder and Executive Director of the *Institute for Responsible Technology* is running the *Campaign for Healthier Eating in America*. He has been communicating to the public on what is happening to our food system and has devoted his career to educating us on what we need to know. You should obtain and watch his movie, *Genetic Roulette, The Gamble of Our Lives*[112]. The information in his movie will turn you towards organic in a second. He also has a couple of powerful books on the subject of GMOs.

Think about how many antibiotics are now being administered to our animals, cows, chickens, fish and pigs, to keep them standing long enough to bring them to market. Why is this? I realize it could partly be the abhorrent conditions these animals are living in. Could what we are feeding them also be partially responsible for how sick they are getting?

The first type of GMO is for corn and cotton when the original organism gets a bacterium gene inserted into its cells. This bacterium is Bt Toxin. They insert this bacterium with a special gun, right into the cell of the product where they want to improve yield.[113]

The advantage of these bacteria in the food is that it has its own insecticide built right into the plant.

We do know that there was dissention by the Monsanto scientists when this product was originally produced. Several scientists spoke out that there was insufficient testing done on the product to allow it to market. These concerns were scrubbed from the original documents and ignored by Michael Taylor, the head of the FDA, Michael Taylor, a former attorney for Monsanto and a future Monsanto VP.[114]

A study called *"A Review on Impacts of Genetically Modified Food on Human Health"* in **The Open Nutraceuticals Journal**, 2011, 4,3-11 3 by Surabhi Nanda, R.K. Singh, R.B. Singh and Sanjay Mishra "Alas, the presence of the toxin in human blood is evidence that this is yet another false assertion that doesn't hold up under closer scrutiny...The GM insecticide toxin is also showing up in fetal blood, which means it could have an impact on future generations, which is exactly what safety advocates like Smith have been warning about."

Jeffry Smith's movie explains that the problem with Bt Toxin is that it pokes holes in insect stomachs, and it is likely that it also pokes holes in human's stomachs.
Roundup Ready® is a trademark of Monsanto Company.

"The subject of the only human-feeding study ever published, wasn't on Bt, it was on the Roundup Ready® soybean. They found that in fact part of that Roundup Ready® gene did transfer to the bacteria living inside human intestines and that these folks had Roundup Ready® gut bacteria. This suggested that the gene, once transferred, continued to function. They didn't follow up to see if the Bt toxin gene also transfers, but this is a critical question. If the toxin-producing gene is in corn chips, for example, and if it then transfers to our gut bacteria, then our intestinal flora become living pesticide factories, producing the Bt toxin over and over again.

An article in Digital Journal called Evidence of GMO toxin absorption and toxicity By E. Hector Corsi May 9, 2012 shows that the latest studies do indeed show that these toxins are being absorbed by the human body causing damage to kidneys, to the liver and is even showing up in human fetus's.[115]

It is a known allergen, it provokes the immune response, it causes digestive issues, it shortens the villi in the stomach, and it causes leaky gut. (Bingo, inflammation and autoimmune disease, no wonder inflammation is growing by leaps and bounds!!!).

Even worse, a new study in the UK has discovered that these toxins continue to be produced in our gut, even when this food has long been digested, continuing to produce its own supply of toxins into our body.[116] [117] [118]

Inserting bacterium into our plants is not part of the natural selection process. There is some feeling that just the insertion and the cloning of the cells does massive damage to the DNA which is, by nature, potentially very harmful to animals and humans.

Genetic Roulette, The Gamble of Our Lives continues

"There is a second type of toxin used for Herbicide tolerance, and this bacterium is inserted into the genes of soy, corn, cotton and sugar beets. The herbicide tolerance bacterium makes the plant "Roundup Ready®" (a trademark of Monsanto Company.)

"Herbicides are supposed to kill the weeds around the plants. A toxin for Herbicide tolerance makes it easier use fewer herbicides in the long run on the plant."

However, "Critics claim that in some cases, the use of herbicide resistant crops can lead to an increase in herbicide use, promote the development of herbicide resistant weeds, and damage biodiversity on the farm. Extensive ecological impact assessments have been addressing these issues."[119]

How safe are GMOs? The only studies, once again, use the same shoddy techniques that were used by the Chemical companies to try and convince us that *Roundup*© was safe. They are studies that are done by the chemical company themselves.

Dr. Russell L. Blaylock, MD in his January 2017 edition of *The Blaylock Wellness Report*:

"A report released by the *Committee for Independent Research and Information on Genetic Engineering* — a nonprofit, independent organization that studies the health effects of GMO food — sheds considerable light on the actions of the food and chemical industry. The committee's report demonstrated potential kidney and liver problems, as well as damage to the heart, adrenal glands, and spleen, as a result of eating genetically modified corn. In tests that favored the food companies, the government regulatory agencies required only a very short-term analysis. The adverse effects of eating GMO foods can take years (even several generations) to fully manifest harmful effects in humans."[120] (Is this absence of evidence or evidence of absence?")

Dr. Blaylock continues "To prevent problems that would occur from being discovered, companies designed tests to their advantage by:

- "Using older animals that die before problems arise
- "Omitting tests on embryos, which are important for pregnant women
- "Testing only a few animals and using obsolete testing methods that weren't sensitive enough to detect damage. Also, as happened with aspartame testing, they ignored the deaths of test animals. Unfortunately, the regulatory agencies have accepted such studies. Here are just a few findings that independent research has uncovered about some of these GMO foods:
    o "Rats fed GMO soy died within three weeks, and mice developed pancreatic and liver problems
    o "Cows mysteriously died when they were fed GMO corn, and many became sterile
    o "When mice were fed GMO potatoes, they developed intestinal damage and bleeding stomachs
    o "Sheep died after grazing in GMO cotton fields."[121]

In an article called ***Dear President-elect Trump: Make America Healthy Again*** by Dr. Edward Group DC, NP, DACBN, DCBCN, DABFM Published on December 15, 2016, Last Updated on December 16, 2016, published by the Global Healing Center, Live Healthy website, he states:

"Simply put, pesticides are poison[122]. And they are everywhere. We use pesticides in our yards, homes, schools, forests, and parks. They permeate our soil, air, and water. Inside our bodies, pesticides disrupt the endocrine system, nervous system, and reproductive system as well as embryonic development. Countless studies link pesticides to Alzheimer's disease, autism spectrum disorders, ADHD, birth defects, and a dozen types of cancer.

"Seven of the most toxic chemical compounds known to man are approved for use as pesticides in the production of food. Organophosphates, commonly used as insecticides, were originally developed by German scientists in World War II as nerve gas. Today, we intentionally spray them on our food."

A scientific journal article called *"A Review on Impacts of Genetically Modified Food on Human Health"* in **The Open Nutraceuticals Journal**, 2011, 4,3-11 3 by Surabhi Nanda, R.K. Singh, R.B. Singh and Sanjay Mishra states:

"GMOS ARE INHERENTLY UNSAFE

"There are several reasons why GM pl*ants* present unique dangers. The first is that the process of genetic engineering itself creates unpredicted alterations, irrespective of which gene is transferred. This creates mutations in and around the insertion site and elsewhere. The biotech industry confidently asserted that gene transfer from GM foods was not possible; the only human feeding study on GM food slater proved that it does take place. The genetic material in soybeans that make them herbicide tolerant transferred into the DNA of human gut bacteria and continued to function. That means that long after we stop eating a GM crop, its foreign GM proteins may be produced inside our intestines."

Dr. Mercola continues: "For example, one 2009 Brazilian study discovered that female rats fed GM soy for 15 months showed significant changes in their uterus and reproductive cycle, compared to rats fed organic soy or those raised without soy. This finding adds to a mounting body of evidence suggesting that GM foods can contribute to a number of reproductive disorders, including: Changes in reproductive hormones, such as excessive production of estrogen, progesterone, follicle stimulating hormone, and luteinizing hormone; Damage to pituitary gland; Retrograde menstruation, in which menstrual discharge travels backwards into the body rather than through the uterus, which can cause a disease known as endometriosis, which may lead to infertility. The disorder can also produce pelvic and leg pain, gastrointestinal problems, chronic fatigue, and a wide variety of other symptoms Testicular changes, including damaged sperm cells"

"Another disturbing study performed by Irina Ermakova with the Russian National Academy of Sciences, reported that more than half the babies from mother rats fed GM soy died within three weeks, while the death rate in the non-GM soy group was only 10 percent. Additionally, the babies in the GM group were smaller, and, worst of all, could not reproduce. In a telling coincidence, after Ermakova's feeding trials were completed, her laboratory started feeding all the rats in the facility commercial rat chow using GM soy. Within two months, the infant mortality facility-wide reached 55 percent ... Unfortunately, you have no way of knowing whether the soy you're eating is genetically modified or not, because GM foods do not have to be labeled as such in the US."

This article appeared in the January 2017 blog on the **Moms Across America** website.[123]

A new study on Glyphosate in the UK was just published. In an article from **GM Watch,**[124] called *Roundup© causes non-alcoholic fatty liver disease at very low doses* by Claire Robinson, she states: "The new peer-reviewed study, led by Dr. Michael Antoniou at King's College London, used cutting-edge profiling methods to describe the molecular composition of the livers of female rats fed an extremely low dose of Roundup, which is based on the chemical glyphosate, over a 2-year period. The dose of glyphosate from the Roundup administered was thousands of times below what is permitted by regulators worldwide."

She continues "The study is the first ever to show a causative link between consumption of Roundup at a real-world environmentally relevant dose and a serious disease.

"Studies that show direct cause carry much more weight with the EPA and global regulatory agencies. This new research could very likely mean the end of Roundup and put a huge dent in GMO chemical farming."

For goodness sake, I hope so!!!! Our lives depend upon it. Of course, when this was written before January 20, 2017 we were all assuming that we were still going to have an active EPA to enforce regulations to protect our health. We will have to wait and see what happens.

There is a notorious French study on rats which were fed a lifetime of GMO corn proved that the rats had a 50-70% chance of developing horrific, grotesque tumors from the diet. Naysayers attempted to refute the science behind the study and a war developed in the scientific community. **Natural News**[125] summarized some findings of the study:

- "Up to 50% of males and 70% of females suffered **premature death**.
- "Rats that drank trace amounts of Roundup (at levels legally allowed in the water supply) had a **200% to 300% increase in large tumors.**
- "Rats fed GM corn and traces of Roundup suffered **severe organ damage** including liver damage and kidney damage.
- "The study fed these rats NK603, the Monsanto variety of GM corn that's grown across North America and widely fed to animals and humans. This is the same corn that's in your corn-based breakfast cereal, corn tortillas, and corn snack chips."

These are the ailments evident in our farm animals that were pointed out in the movie *Genetic Roulette, The Gamble Of Our Lives*. I can't prove that these ailments are directly correlated to the animals eating GMOs, but just the thought that GMO's could be responsible, makes me want to take a precautionary stance.

- Gastrointestinal
- Accelerated aging
- Immune issues
- Reproductive issues
- Insulin and Cholesterol issues
- Asthma
- Allergies[126] [127]
- Headaches
- Fatigue
- Diabetes
- Liver and kidney issues
- Organ damage
- Cancer
- Skin issues
- Brain fog

- Depression
- Aggression
- High Blood Pressure
- Heart disease
- Cancer
- MS
- Obesity
- Infant mortality
- Parkinson's disease[128]
- Alzheimer's disease[129]
- Autism[130] [131]

When genetically modified foods are removed from the animal's diet, their health conditions seem to improve in as little as three days. Same with humans, doctors are finding that when genetically modified foods are removed from human diets, health also improved[132].

"Other organs may be affected too, such as the heart and spleen, or blood cells," stated the paper. In fact, some of the animals fed genetically modified organisms had altered body weights, which is "a very good predictor of side effects in various organs."[133]

I understand these are observational results. Until recently there have been no scientific studies made public that support this. The studies that have been done are squashed, the scientists are silenced or lose their jobs, and their research is destroyed. So, as a result, we are back to the "absence of evidence, vs. evidence of absence." How the animals are responding – in my opinion, is the evidence. At least it is enough proof for me.

Brazil's National Council for Food and Nutrition Security just published a document citing 750 studies that show the environmental and health risks that are being ignored by countries regulatory agencies, in a lengthy report recently published in **GM Watch, 2/27/2017 *The 750 studies that GMO regulatory bodies often ignore.*** "Credibility damaging campaigns for researches and authors mentioning such hazards and uncertainties are also described."[134] "In the section on health risks, the book's authors note that the scientific literature shows 'immune and allergic reactions' in animals and humans to Bt toxins of the type engineered into GM Bt plants.[135]"

The herbicides get absorbed in the crop. The insertion process damages the DNA and causes mutations. In corn, the process also switches on an allergen.

There is also some discussion that a new pathogen is being born after GMO use that could have long-term implications.[136]

Also, it is possible that as an antibiotic Roundup not only kills external bacteria, it also kills our good gut bacteria. Unfortunately it does not appear to kill bad gut bacteria.[137] A double whammy.

GMOs are also an endocrine disruptor.[138] [139]

In soy, (90% of our soy is now GMO) it turns off a Trypsin inhibitor. Trypsin inhibitors are important to digestion.[140] [141]

GMOs interfere with the production of serotonin (the feel-good hormone) and melatonin (the sleep hormone.)[142]

I just read an article where **Monsanto** cotton seed, sold in India, destroyed crops by attracting a new type of bug that the farmers had never dealt with previously. The article was discussing all of the Indian farmers who were committing suicide because they lost their entire crops. The Indian government is now involved in the issue.[143] The field workers in India were also suffering from terrible skin conditions. When Water Buffalo were allowed to feed on the plants after harvest in these fields, they died within 24 hours.

Isn't that astonishing? Sadly, it makes sense to me.

"There are also reports of negative results and illness from Liberty Glusofinate© by Bayer.[144]" This is what the label of Liberty Glusofinate states:[145] (The warnings on Roundup© by Monsanto are very similar).

"If swallowed

- "Rinse mouth thoroughly with plenty of water.
- "Do not induce vomiting.
- "Get medical attention immediately.

"If in Eyes

- "Hold eye open and rinse slowly and gently with water for 15-20 minutes
- "Remove contact lenses, if present, after the first 5 minutes, then continue "rinsing eye.
- "Get medical attention if irritation develops or persists.

"If on skin or clothing

- "Take off contaminated clothing.
- "Wash skin immediately with plenty of soap and water.
- "Get medical attention.

"If inhaled

- "Move person to fresh air.
- "Get medical attention if breathing difficulty develops"

And they want us to eat food that has had this sprayed on it?

There have also been human health issues when Bt toxin was sprayed over fields in Washington State and Oregon.[146]

When sheep in Warangal District, Andhra Pradesh were allowed to graze on the remnants of the cotton in the fields they showed signs of disease within the first 3 days. Mortality occurred within 1 week.[147]

Twelve dairy cows died after being fed GM maize and silage. This happened on a farm in Woelfersheim in the state of Hesse, Germany.[148]

Farmers in Germany reported that their livestock became sterile after eating Bt corn.[149]

There is a study by Judy Carman, PhD published in the peer reviewed journal Organic Systems about a study with pigs[150]. Pigs that ate GMO feed were compared to pigs that were not fed a GMO diet. The pigs on the GMO diet showed lots of health issues that are a cause of concern:

"Scientists randomized and fed isowean pigs either a mixed GM soy and GM corn (maize) diet for approximately 23 weeks (nothing out of the ordinary for most pigs in the United States), which is unfortunately the normal lifespan of a commercial pig from weaning to slaughter. Equal numbers of male and female pigs were present in each group. The GM diet was associated with gastric and uterine differences in pigs. GM pigs had uteri that were 25% heavier than non-GM fed pigs. GM-fed pigs had a higher rate of severe stomach inflammation with a rate of 32% compared to 125 of non-GM fed pigs."[151]

Another study available that prove this point is a French research paper on the effects of GMO corn fed to rats.[152]

There are known environmental detrements to GMO crops.

"Unintended harm to other organisms: pollen from B.t. corn caused high mortality rates in monarch butterfly caterpillars. Monarch caterpillars consume milkweed pl*ants*, not corn, but the fear is that pollen from B.t. corn is blown by the wind onto milkweed pl*ants* in neighboring fields, the caterpillars could eat the pollen and perish. B.t. toxins kill many species of insect larva." This toxin is killing both good and bad insects, i.e. bees which are critical to our crop pollination.

Moms Across America has a website with Mom's testimonials that their kids get better when they stop eating genetically modified organisms. Take a look.[153] The leader of the group felt so strongly about this issue that she went to **The Hague International Court** hearing about **Monsanto** at **The Hague** in Europe in November 2016. This group w*ants* to save our children. ***And we need to act now.***

All of these substances are killing both the good and the bad bugs. They are wiping out our bee population. No bees, no pollinati*on* of our crops, no crops.

Europe has banned many of these substances. A scientific report on the dangers of GMOs leaked to the public, some years ago, and the public immediately responded by not buying the GMO food.[154] Companies like **Unilever, Nestle, McDonald,** and **Burger King** in Europe immediately responded BUT ONLY IN EUROPE. (Recently parts of this ban were lifted, so Europeans will now have the same consequences of GMO crops as the rest of the world.)[155]

So, what do we do here in the US? It's been difficult to get the word out because anyone who speaks out about GMOs is demonized. It is also difficult to get the word out because anyone who speaks out against the herbicides and insecticides being sprayed on our crops is also being demonized. Industry-sponsored research is rigged. GMOs and herbicides and insecticides are protected by our government agencies and our Congress. (I think, too much money, honey)

Chemical companies push the concept that their food grown with toxins is "feeding the world."[156]

"Feeding the world" is always a future based "goal" never to be obtained any time soon. GMOs have been on the market since 1996. When are they going to feed the world? The answer is never because that's not what they are intended to do. I've heard an estimate of 80% of the GMOs grown in the US is used for force-feeding factory farmed animals. [157]

USA today reported, "It takes about 15 pounds of feed to make 1 pound of beef, 6 pounds of feed for 1 pound of pork and 5 pounds of feed for 1 pound of chicken."

In January 2015, the *Independent Science News* reported that "researchers from Iowa have shown that organic farming methods can yield almost as highly as pesticide-intensive methods. Other researchers, from Berkeley, California, have reached a similar conclusion."[158]

I have also read that we have plenty of food to feed the world. The problem is that we don't have appropriate distribution channels. The other problem is that many people cannot afford food, whether it is GMO or not. Perhaps that should be where our focus is, instead of on GMO soy and corn.

Still, the non-GMO movement is growing. Whole food stated that GMO verified products were up 15% the first year and 30% the second year. **BUY GMO VERIFIED.**

Any drop-in Market share will find our food companies responding. In the meantime, be vigilant and only buy organic. Jeffry Smith believes that if there is a 5% change,[159] just 5%, more companies will start to swing to organically grown vegetables and fruits. Vote with your dollars.

The Institute for Responsible Technology has a guide of products that are GMO safe. The link is noted below. You can download their printed guide.

There is also an article at **RealFarmacy.com** called *"400 Companies That DO Not Use GMOs."*[160]

Weston Price Organization has an article on their website called **4 *Tips To Avoid GMO*s**[161] March 30, 2009, written by Jerry Smith. These four things are pretty simple to embrace:

1. Buy Organic
2. Look for Non-GMO Labels
3. Avoid at risk Ingredients
4. Get a copy of the Institute for Responsible Technology Shopping Guide, and use it.

The good news is that Millennials are demanding transparency and they want non-GMO foods. Within ten years, they will be 75% of the workforce in the US.[162] They will be the bulk of the spending population; they will get attention, and they will be heard. (This article has disappeared on-line – how interesting. I saved a copy on my computer.)

It doesn't make sense to me, science or no science, that eating herbicides and insecticides could possibly be healthy for the body whether we are talking about animals or talking about humans.

Remember, these plants have been modified in a way that could have never happened in nature, to make the crop what is known as "Roundup Ready®" (a trademark of Monsanto Company.)

Roundup© was discussed above as one of the many toxins being sprayed on our conventional crops.

What else can you do? Buy grass-fed grass-finished beef and organic milk, yogurt and butter (or ghee) from pastured cows. Buy pastured chickens and pastured chicken eggs. You will also avoid hormones, steroids, and antibiotics this way. Meat, fish, and chicken will be discussed further in **Factory farmed meat, chicken and fish and good alternatives**, Part 3, Chapter 14 in my food section.

I just re-watched the ***Genetic Roulette*** Movie. What I missed the first time I watched that was the statement that Monsanto *wants* to own all of the seeds for all of the crops in the world. We can't let that happen. We all must get involved. If they are allowed to do that, my fear is it could end mankind. My opinion.

A new article published just a few weeks ago – by **Eco Watch**, January 4, 2017, by John Roulac, ***Spaceship Earth, Your Main Oxygen Systems Are Collapsing***[163] discusses an overlooked, but the devastating result of our factory farming methods that had not even occurred to me.

"... an imminent loss of oxygen just happens to be a current fact, because the ocean's phytoplankton (which provides two-thirds of the planet's oxygen) is rapidly dying off. Industrial agriculture not only contaminates our oceans with pesticide and nitrogen fertilizer runoff, leading to massive dead zones; it is stripping our soils of carbon, which ends up in the oceans and creates acidification. At the current trajectory, in just a few decades there won't be much left alive in our oceans as the phytoplankton dies — all because of how we grow our food."

The New York Times also warned of the dying of our oceans in its article *"Our Deadened, Carbon-Soaked Seas"* by Richard W. Spinrad, chief scientist at the National Oceanic and Atmospheric Administration, and Ian Boyd, chief scientific adviser to the British government's Department for Environment, Food, and Rural Affairs. October 15, 2015 the article states: "Ocean and coastal waters around the world are beginning to tell a disturbing story. The seas, like a sponge, are absorbing increasing amounts of carbon dioxide from the atmosphere, so much so that the chemical balance of our oceans and coastal waters is changing and posing a growing threat to marine ecosystems. Over the past 200 years, the world's seas have absorbed more than 150 billion metric tons of carbon from human activities. This is known as ocean acidification; this process makes it difficult for shellfish, corals, and other marine organisms to grow and reproduce."

Food for thought and a request for action: if we even want to have a planet, we need to stop this.

My final thoughts on the subject:

Monsanto has done studies to prove that **Roundup**© is safe and that GMO's are safe. I have no idea what's real and what's Memorex. I choose to proceed with caution. I am avoiding these chemicals as much as I possibly can. Do your own research and make your own decisions.

I believe that eliminating pesticides and GMO foods has personally helped me find wellness again.

Be informed. Get involved.

Chapter 7

Toxins in our processed food and fast food

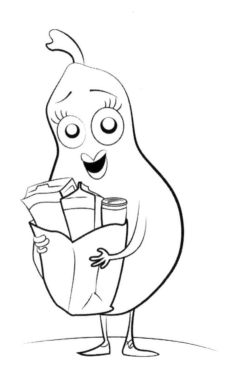

Dousing the flame of inflammation:

THE BIG TAKEAWAYS ON PROCESSED FOOD AND FAST FOOD

- Processed food and fast food are both filled with chemicals, non-foods, GMOs, sugar, and salt, and they are designed to be addictive and make you fat.
- There are few ingredients in these products that nourish your body.
- If you can't pronounce ingredients on the label, don't buy it.
- Processed foods and Fast food cause inflammation
- It is important to cook real food at home.
- Cooking doesn't have to be complicated to feed your body real nutrients.

"You are what you eat, so don't be fast, cheap, easy, or fake."

JONATHAN KARPATHIOS[165]

"Maybe we should stop asking why real food is so expensive, and start asking why processed food is so cheap"

FOOD MATTERS

"... you are literally what you eat physically ... So, if you are eating junk, if you are eating toxins, or if you're eating heavy metals, your body, your brains, your organs, and your skin, and everything that's in your physical body becomes junk, becomes toxic, and becomes processed."

MIKE ADAMS, AKA **THE HEALTH RANGER** FROM **THE TRUTH ABOUT CANCER**

I have a simple rule with processed food. If I can't pronounce the ingredients, I don't buy or eat it.

Last year I purchased a book called **Pandora's Lunchbox** Scribner, a Division of Simon and Schuster, Inc. 2013 by Melanie Warner. I strongly recommend you read it even though the book totally freaked me out. Melanie was a food editor for the New York Times and got curious about why much of our food doesn't rot. This statement from the back of her book explains "If a piece of individually wrapped cheese can retain its shape, color, and texture for years, what does it say about the food we eat and feed to our children?" The book takes a close investigative look at research labs, university food science departments, and the factories that are developing our food. The book opens at a convention of cheap fake food products available for Big Food to use instead of real food ingredients. These fake food products taste good and are addictive. And they have no food value. Yikes!

"Warner looks at how decades of food science have resulted in the cheapest, most abundant, most addictive and most nutritionally inferior food in the world, and uncovers startling evidence about the profound health implications of the packaged and Fast Foods that we are eating on a daily basis."

The other problem with processed food and fast food is that they are loaded with MSG. Most people, I think, are aware of the dire effects on the body from MSG, but they are not aware that it has been rebranded under a multitude of names to hide that fact that it is still being put into our food.

Dr. Frank Lipman, MD stated in his blog **No More MSG: The Food Additive You Should Learn Live Without** Mar 12, 2013 "Processed foods fill the body with additives. Whole foods don't. MSG, which is found in an estimated 80% of processed foods, sets off a variety of adverse reactions such as skin rashes, headaches, moodiness, irritability, IBS, heart palpitations, depression and more, depending on your tolerance. How fast and hard you get hit by these problems depends on your ability to tolerate it, but regardless, eating foods laced with MSG are devastating to your organs. In short, MSG can make people feel lousy in the short term and potentially, very, very sick in the long-term."[166]

Check the labels for these names[167]. (They are all different terms for MSG.)

- Glutamic Acid (E 620)2
- Glutamate (E 620)
- Monosodium Glutamate (E 621)

- Monopotassium Glutamate (E 622)
- Calcium Glutamate (E 623)
- Monoammonium Glutamate (E 624)
- Magnesium Glutamate (E 625)
- Natrium Glutamate
- Yeast Extract
- Anything hydrolyzed
- Any hydrolyzed protein
- Calcium Caseinate
- Sodium Caseinate
- Yeast Food
- Yeast Nutrient
- Autolyzed Yeast
- Gelatin
- Textured Protein
- Soy Protein Isolate
- Whey Protein Isolate
- Anything: protein
- Vetsin
- Ajinomoto

Names of ingredients that often contain or produce processed free glutamic acid (MSG)

- Carrageenan (E 407)
- Bouillon and broth
- Stock
- Any flavors or flavoring
- Maltodextrin
- Citric Acid, Citrate (E 330)
- Anything ultra-pasteurized
- Barley malt
- Pectin (E 440)
- Protease
- Anything enzyme modified
- Anything containing enzymes

- Malt extract
- Soy sauce
- Soy sauce extract
- Anything protein fortified
- Seasonings

I read once in a different article that "Natural flavors" on a label is also suspect as a cover for MSG.

Glutamic acid found in unadulterated "whole food" protein does not cause adverse reactions. To cause adverse reactions, the glutamic acid must have been processed/manufactured or come from protein that has been fermented.

Avoiding MSG is critical if you want to heal your inflammation, so you need to be vigilant.

Our bodies need real food and nutrients to function. So, in case you are curious about what is going on with our health in the United States, and why disease is rampant, it is because we are eating fake food that gives our body nothing to survive.

Dr. Joseph Mercola OD, (Doctor of Osteopathic Medicine) breaks processed foods down to the following issues, in his article **9 Ways That Eating Processed Food Made the World Sick and Fat:** (2/12/2014)[168]

1. "They are loaded with sugar or corn syrup.
2. "They are loaded with salt.
3. "They are designed to make you fat.
4. "They are designed to be addictive.
5. "They are loaded with preservatives, artificial ingredients, and artificial food dyes.
6. "They are particularly high in refined carbohydrates.
7. "They are very low in nutrients.
8. "They are very low in fiber.
9. "It takes less time to digest processed foods. The brain doesn't register that it ate at all and it *wants* MORE." (Sugar has this effect on the body too. See my discussion of sugar, Part 3, Chapter 8.)
10. "Some of the chemicals in the processed food are carcinogens.

11. "These foods are often loaded with bad fats, the Trans fats.
12. "More than 70% of processed foods carry genetically modified ingredients.[169]"

Many processed foods are engineered to be very rewarding to the brain, making you want to eat more and more.[170]

In an article by **NHS**, *Eating Processed Foods*, they give examples of processed foods:[171]

- Breakfast cereals
- Cheese
- Canned vegetables
- Bread
- Savory snacks, such as crisps
- Meat products, such as bacon
- "Convenience foods," such as microwave meals or ready meals
- Drinks, such as milk or soft drinks

Most deli meats, bacon, cheeses, frozen foods, all fall into this category. READ THE INGREDIENTS. If you can't pronounce it or if it is outside the guidelines below, avoid this food:

Total fat[172]
High: more than 17.5g of fat per 100g
Low: 3g of fat or less per 100g

Saturated fat
High: more than 5g of saturated fat per 100g
Low: 1.5g of saturated fat or less per 100g

Sugars
High: more than 22.5g of total sugars per 100g
Low: 5g of total sugars or less per 100g

Salt
High: more than 1.5g of salt per 100g (or 0.6g sodium)
Low: 0.3g of salt or less per 100g (or 0.1g sodium)

Also, the **National Institute of Health** just published a study in November 2016 ***"Food additives promote inflammation, colon cancer in mice"*** that finds a direct link of food emulsifiers in processed foods to inflammation and cancer in mice.[173]

"Dietary emulsifiers, which are chemically similar to detergents, are added to many processed foods to improve texture and extend shelf life. Their use is regulated and monitored by the U.S. Food and Drug Administration. Recent research, however, suggests that some emulsifiers might affect gut microbes in unexpected ways, at least in animals. Scientists at Georgia State University previously found that mice fed low levels of common dietary emulsifiers developed altered gut microbiota and a thinned mucus barrier protecting the lining of their intestines. The mice also developed low-grade intestinal inflammation and metabolic syndrome — which are conditions that increase the risk of Type II diabetes, heart disease, and stroke."

"There is no such thing as junk food. There is junk and there is food."

UNKNOWN

One more thing, this article from the New York Times, ***The Extraordinary Science of Addictive Junk Food*** 2/24/2013,[174] should be mandatory reading. It clearly shows how we, the public, have been manipulated by Big Food, and how they knowingly have changed their products to make us unhealthy and fat. They took no responsibility for their actions and were fully aware of what the results would be.

I do buy some processed food, but it is limited.

I buy organic lunch meat; I buy **Applegate Farms** lunch meat and bacon.

I am sensitive to dairy, so I don't buy cheese, but check ingredients – you may want to eat dairy, but read my chapter about dairy (Part 3, Chapter 12) before you buy it. Watch the sugar, and buy full fat. Buy organic pastured dairy.

I buy **Rao's Spaghetti Sauce**; it's pretty clean.

I read the labels on everything before I buy it. If there are ingredients I can't pronounce, I don't buy it. I carefully monitor that amount of sugar in the item, by serving. Remember, 4 grams of sugar equals one teaspoon.

It feels too good to feel good to not be vigilant.

The bottom line is that you need to COOK real food at home. It doesn't have to be complicated; it just has to feed your body what it needs and *wants*. I have listed my favorite cookbooks on my website to get you started. www.cherylmhealthmuse. com. They are listed under resources.

I eat Paleo, which means that other than organic vegetables, I eat no dairy and I do eat pastured meats. If I can't get to the farmers' market during a certain week, I have farm fresh vegetables delivered in the middle of the night from a local farm. If I need something in a pinch, I go to **Whole Foods** or **Sprouts** (or **Erewhon** or **Mothers**, which are a bit of a distance away.) (Find your organic food market in your own area.) If you want to tame the inflammation and put your autoimmune condition at bay, you can figure this all out.

If you need ideas, follow me on Facebook.

Cooking can be as simple as steaming a head of cauliflower, throwing it into your blender or *Vitamix*, adding a little almond milk, a bit of ghee, and a touch of sea salt and turning it on. Walla, soup. That is just as fast as microwaving a frozen entrée.

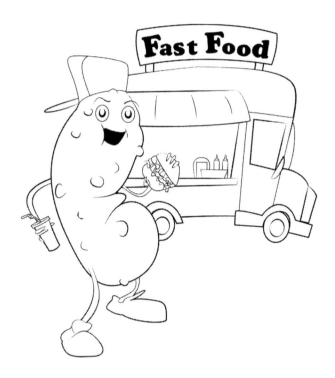

FAST FOOD

"Your body doesn't have the ability to turn garbage into a high-quality product. All your cells, muscles, skin, bones, etc. are built by the food that you supply. Choose wisely"

NUTRITION AMLIFEIED.COM

You are what you eat.

Just like processed food, fast food, in most instances, gives you absolutely no food nutrients, so what do you expect your body to live on?

Before I got sick, I often asked myself, on the rare occasion that I ate fast food, how they could make it so cheap.

From pink goop (which I think they don't use anymore) to other concoctions of chemicals and fake foods that simulate food taste, texture, and color plus the preservatives that keep it from rotting, no wonder we are all getting fat and sick.

I will grant you that it is fast and easy, and takes no thought or planning. But other than an occasional **Chipotle** which is organic, and non-GMO, I am thriving and doing just fine not eating fast food anymore.

Let's talk about the other hazards, and then I will give suggestions on what I do when I am traveling, or out and about away from home, and I need food.

The Official Site For the Stay At Home Mom breaks down the risks to the following 5 points[175] in an article called **Your Kids Become What You Feed Them – 7 Dangers of Fast Food**:

1. "Obesity – Just one Fast Food meal can have all of the calories and fat that you need for your entire day. There is also hidden sugar in these foods.

2. "Risk of Diabetes – since you are eating way more calories than you need at one meal, and since it is laden with bad fat, your risk of Diabetes goes up significantly

3. "Risk of Stroke – between the bad fats that clog your arteries, and the high salt level in the foods, you become a ticking time bomb for a stroke.

4. "Risk of Heart Attack – same problem as above, but instead of blocking blood to your brain, the excess fat and salt block blood to your heart.

5. "Real nutrients are limited in fast food. Since the body is starving for nutrients, and since it processes all of these fake ingredients quickly, right after eating a big meal of fast food, the body screams MORE."

The article concludes "Taking the little extra time to buy fresh food from the grocery store and cook a meal at home will save you money in the long run. You will get more food for your buck, plus you won't have to pay medical bills down the road."

Ingredients in Fast Food according to an article in **Positive Med**[176] called *10 Disgusting Facts About Fast Food* April 20, 2013:

These are some of the "yummy, aarrggh" ingredients in fast food

- **"McDonalds** Milkshake has 50 chemicals in it to imitate the flavor of real strawberry
- "Fast foods healthiest choice, salad, has an antifreeze chemical on it which causes eye and skin irritation
- "A can of **Coca Cola** has ten teaspoons of sugar. They add other chemicals so that you don't vomit after drinking.
- "Cheese used in fast food is only 49% cheese. The rest is chemicals. So, ½ of the food is not real
- "Chicken nuggets are approximately 50 percent skeletal muscle, with the remainder composed primarily of fat, with some blood vessels and nerve present. Higher-power views showed generous quantities of epithelium and associated supportive tissue including squamous epithelium from skin or vice versa."[177]

You want non-food? Yuck!

All of these factors exasperate your inflammation.

You must learn to eat clean, and that means traveling with real food from home.

- When I am out and about, I always have green apples with me. I buy **Justin's** almond butter packets so that with the apple I have a fulfilling treat.
- I carry protein bars that are low in sugar and high in protein. (I am diabetic, so I need to make sure I have healthy fuel to keep my blood sugar steady.)
- If I am out and about, and not close to home, I stop at a **Sprouts** or a **Whole Foods** and buy **Applegate** organic cold cuts, and a head of lettuce, and make an instant wrap. It takes just a couple of minutes more than going through a drive through.
- I buy **Vital Farm's** pasture raised chicken eggs, and hard boil them so that I have them handy when I am out and about.

- I buy Cassava Chips by **Artisan Tropic** and eat them instead of potato chips, and I can easily carry them when I am on the road. (Potatoes have over 35 pesticides and herbicides on them)[178]
- I buy organic nuts, and keep them in my purse for a little pick me up.

In other words, I don't allow myself to be in a situation where the only food that is available is fast food. When we don't have healthy choices available, we make bad decisions that interfere with our wellness.

Since we are getting so sick as a population, some clever food people are trying to fill the gap and do healthy fast food. It's coming in the future. I read an article about a fast food joint in Florida that used organic produce and grass fed beef, (**Rainforest Café**)[179] and had lines out the door and around the block. There is a fast food restaurant in the Bay Area in California, called the **Organic Coop** that uses **Mary's organic chicken**, which they fry in coconut oil. Even the bun is organic.

It's starting to happen, so keep the faith. But, in the meantime, plan ahead.

AVOID PROCESSED FOOD. READ THE LABELS. AVOID FAST FOOD. IT'S KILLING YOU!

Chapter 8

Sugar makes us sick

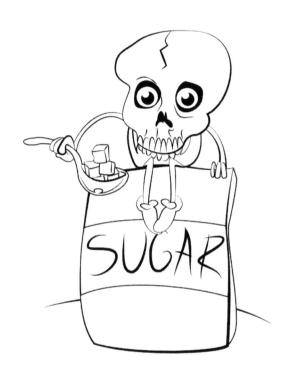

Dousing the flame of inflammation:

THE BIG TAKEAWAYS ON SUGAR

- Sugar is horrific on the body.
- Sugar is sugar is sugar. Fructose is the worst, but Maple Syrup, Agave, and Honey have the same effect on the body.
- Sugar substitutes (pink packet, yellow packet, blue packet) are pure chemicals and interrupt body functions while offering no food value. These chemical sweeteners cause leaky gut. They are a source of inflammation. Stevia and brown rice syrup are the exception and a few sugar alcohols (some people react negatively to these) are also ok.
- Sugar is linked to many diseases and is one of the leading causes of inflammation.
- You need to detox off of sugar, which is a drug worse than cocaine, and then watch sugar intake in the future to cure your inflammation.

This one is tough, but if you bear with me, and detox off the sugar, you will feel better, a lot better. Sugar fuels the fire of your inflammation, so it's crucial that you reduce your sugar intake dramatically.

And sugar is toxic, so this is critical.

In a review in the New York Times *"What Not to Eat: 'The Case Against Sugar'"* Jan 2, 2017, By Dan Barber, he states: "Gary Taubes begins with a kick in the teeth in his just-published book **The Case Against Sugar** Alfred A. Knopf (December 27, 2016). Sugar is not only the root cause of today's diabetes and obesity epidemics (had these been infectious diseases, the Centers for Disease Control and Prevention would have long ago declared an emergency), but also, according to Taubes, is probably related to heart disease, hypertension, many common cancers and Alzheimer's."

Dan Barber continues that "Taubes's writing is both inflammatory and copiously researched. It is also well timed. In September, a researcher at the University of California, San Francisco, uncovered documents showing that Big Sugar paid three Harvard scientists in the 1960s to play down the connection between sugar and heart disease and instead point the finger at saturated fat. Coca-Cola and candy makers made similar headlines for their forays into nutrition science, funding studies that discounted the link between sugar and obesity."

According to Dr. Mark Hyman MD, as a nation, we eat 152 lbs. each of sugar a year.[181] Wow!

Dr. Hyman continues: "We should be eating no more than 6-9 teaspoons of sugar a day, but instead are consuming 22 teaspoons of sugar as an adult, and 34 teaspoons of sugar as kids. Your body wasn't meant to handle more than two teaspoons of sugar a day, so even the 6-9 teaspoon guideline is a lot.

"The biggest culprit is soda, but amazingly enough, fruit juices have the same amount of sugar in them that soda does. We just drink more sugar.

"Also, we eat 146 lbs. of flour in a year, which converts to sugar."

So, what harm does sugar do to the body?

According to Sarah Wilson, author of *"I Quit Sugar":* Clarkson Potter (April 8, 2014)

"Sugar Makes Us Sick."

"There is a direct correlation and causal effect on the body for

- "Heart Disease
- "Cancer
- "Diabetes
- "Tooth decay
- "Hypertension
- "Insomnia
- "Dizziness
- "Allergies
- "Hair loss
- "Alzheimer's

"Skin issues "In addition:

- "It ages the body and adds wrinkles.
- "It increases uric acid which causes kidney disease.
- "It creates fatty liver.

- "It interferes with Thyroid function and makes it sick.
- "It causes hormone imbalances impacting cortisol and sex hormones.
- "It interferes with our appetite and makes us fat.
- "And most important IT CAUSES INFLAMMATION by doing havoc in the digestive track. It ruins your gut flora."

Sugar messes with our appetite hormones, Leptin and Ghrelin. Since it has no food value, your body craves nutrients and keeps asking for more, and the addiction to sugar causes the body to never be satisfied with enough.

Before I detoxed off of sugar, I recognized that I was always hungry, no matter how much I ate; I didn't understand that this was created by eating sugar. I had no turn-off switch with food and gained lots of weight.

When we eat sugar and fructose, it goes to the liver, and since it can't be used for energy, it gets stored as fat. Liver stores it and insulin is produced. Sugar is the cause of high Triglycerides.[182] Fructose damages 500 genes that are related to brain function and memory.[183]

Glucose which is created from complex carbohydrates and protein is good for us. When we eat glucose, it goes into the cells in the body and gets utilized for energy.

Sugar addiction includes cane sugar, glucose, sucrose, fructose, lactose, and maltose. Sugar is sugar is sugar. No matter what form it comes in. Agave is one of the worst; Corn Syrup, cane sugar, honey maple syrup are all sugar. Molasses is not far behind.

Be careful of the sugar alcohols, sugars that end with itol, xylitol, sorbitol and mannitol. The impact of the body for sugar is significantly reduced, but for me, they are an immediate cause of diarrhea. Not a good look. Completely avoid all of the chemical sweeteners, Equal, Sweet and Low, Saccharin, Splenda, etc. They each have diverse effects on the body, and the chemicals are poison.

According to Dr. Mark Hyman, MD., artificial sweeteners lead to weight gain. They slow metabolism, interfere with the brain, and cause our body temperatures to drop. We eat 24 pounds of artificial sweeteners a year. And they are a cause of diabetes.[184]

Furthermore, they interfere with our digestive system and are a cause of leaky gut.

Better choices for sweetness are stevia (I have found that the best is from **Trader Joe's**, get the 100% pure variety) and rice malt syrup. Coconut milk, sweet potato, and cinnamon are also better options.

And it is addictive; sugar is eight times as addictive as cocaine;[185] it lights up the same place in the brain as cocaine. So, it's an addiction that is hard to detox off of, and there are withdrawal symptoms.

So, how do you detox off of sugar?

Detoxing off of sugar means eliminating processed foods and fast foods, which are both loaded, in most cases, with sugar. So, cooking becomes non-negotiable. (Cooking is how you are going to provide your body with all of the beautiful nutrients that it needs anyway, so this is just one more reason to cook!)

Detoxing off of sugar can be difficult. I got sick like I had the flu, my body ached, I had cold sweats, and my moods were up and down. It wasn't fun. And I started detoxing immediately, probably because of the amount of sugar I was eating. For me, it only took ten days to come out the other side. For others, it sometimes takes four weeks before the withdrawal symptoms to even begin. It varies by person. I have read 30 days, I have read two weeks I have read six weeks, but however long it takes for you, it is freeing to be on the other side. In no longer than six weeks, appetite changes and gets on a natural cycle. Now eating minimal sugar, my appetite is diminished, my blood sugar is more stable (I have Type II Diabetes), and I am happier. There is food freedom. There is emotional wellness. My mood swings are gone. I no longer crave sugar, and it is easy for me to pass on desserts when I am out with friends. After reviewing the list of risks from eating sugar, it was well worth the ten days it took for me to break the addiction to the stuff. If it takes you six weeks, trust me, it is still worth it. When you come out the other end of a sugar detox, the addiction is gone.

In a recent opinion column in the **New York Times** by David Leonhardt *A Month Without Sugar* 12/30/2016, having taken up the sugar challenge, he writes:[186]

"If you give up sugar for a month, you'll become part of a growing anti-sugar movement. Research increasingly indicates that an overabundance of simple carbohydrates and sugar, in particular, is the No. 1 problem in modern diets. An aggressive, well-financed campaign by the sugar industry masked this reality for years. Big Sugar instead placed the blame on fats — which seem, after all, as if they should cause obesity.

"But fats tend to have more nutritional value than sugar, and sugar is far easier to overeat. Put it this way: Would you find it easier to eat two steaks or two pieces of cake?"

"Most public authorities think everybody would be healthier eating less sugar," says Marion Nestle of N.Y.U. "There is tons of evidence."[187]

"The sugar that occurs naturally in fruit, vegetables and dairy is allowed." Nobody eats too much of those, ..." Nestle says, "... not with the fiber and vitamins and minerals they have."[188]

When you are done with the detox, your skin will be dramatically improved, and interestingly enough, my sense of smell became acute. I can smell sugar now as I walk down aisles at the grocery store. The smell is overwhelming.

It is a significant step in ending your body pain and healing your gut.

So, how would you take the challenge and detox off of sugar?

1. Read food labels. If there are hidden sugars in the food, toss them out. You will be eliminating most boxed foods, most canned foods, most processed foods. And for the period of the detox, no grains.

2. Grocery shop so that you have great choices on hand while you are doing the detox. Try not to eat out. It is much easier to control what goes into your food if you prepare it yourself.

3. Eat veggies, but for the time of the detox avoid sweet potatoes, potatoes, squash, and beets. Stay away from starchy vegetables

4. Eat fats. Vitamins A, E, K, B are all fat-soluble vitamins, and you need fat for your body to utilize them
   a) Nuts and seeds
   b) Olive oil
   c) Coconut oil
   d) Avocado
   e) Wild caught fresh fish, like salmon

5. Eat protein

6. For snacks, try guacamole and celery sticks. The celery satisfies your desire to chomp. The guacamole is always a lovely treat and avocado is a good fat. MAKE YOUR OWN. There are hidden sugars in salsas.

7. The only juices that I drank when I did my detox were pomegranate and cranberry, no sugar. I bought them at Trader Joes, but I know there are some other brands. A little of one of these juices in filtered water with a drop of stevia is a lovely treat.

8. Organic Berries and green apples are the only fruits you should eat during your sugar detox. Fresh blueberries (Blueberries are very low in sugar) Raspberries are also a good choice. Buy organic apples and berries since non-organic are laden with pesticides and herbicides. If fresh are not available, buy frozen organic blueberries and raspberries.

9. Green apples are a great choice. I love Granny Smith and Pippins when in season. Winesaps are also a good choice. A good sour apple is a great treat.

10. Drink **PGX** fiber powder when you first get up. Mix it with water and drink it quickly before it sets.

11. Take a good multi-vitamin

12. Take Chromium, essential for body function.

13. Carry an emergency kit with you
    a) **Arsana** almond butter packets
    b) Nuts
    c) Salmon jerky
    d) Turkey jerky
    e) Can of wild salmon
    f) Fresh blueberries (Blueberries are very low in sugar)

14. Use full-fat Dairy. When food companies take the fat out, sugar goes in. For Milk and yogurt, you want full fat. There are other reasons to drink full-fat, which we will discuss in the Chapter 12 on Dairy, if you can, eliminate dairy completely for the period of the detox.

15. Eliminate all grains for the period of the detox. By doing this, you have also eliminated gluten.

16. Eliminate sauces (loaded with hidden sugars.) Careful of condiments. Ketchup and mustards are often loaded with sugar.

17. Eat savory breakfasts. Eggs are a great choice. (add in a handful of spinach, and some green onions and mushrooms to change it up)

18. Breathe. See my chapter on stress for my favorite breathing exercise, by Dr. Andrew Weil.

19. Get 8 hours of sleep.

Once you have come down off of your sugar addiction, stay conscious of how much sugar you are eating. Be careful that you don't retrigger your sugar addiction.

Suggestions[189]:

- My favorite thing that I read somewhere is that you eat like it's 1934[190]. (Sounds like it could be a song). Our grandparents didn't eat processed, fast, or sugar laden foods.
- Shop the edges of the grocery store.
- Eat the entire fruit. You need the fiber, and with the fiber, it is more filling.
- I found two phrases I love
    o JERF – Just Eat Real Food[191] and
    o KISS – Keep it Simple Stupid[192]

- Learn to read the labels on the food you eat. Even a carton of plain yogurt has six teaspoons of sugar in it. Note portion sizes. If a carton has two servings and 20 grams of sugar, that is 20 grams x 2 or 40 grams, which equals ten teaspoons of sugar.
- The best bread to eat is sourdough. It is fermented, so it's good for blood sugar, it has minimal gluten and sugar in it. (the fermenting process utilizes the sugar)
- A couple of sugar swaps suggested by JJ Virgin, another guru on sugar, from her UTube presentation *Simple Sugar Swaps*[193]:

  a) "For raisins, use blueberries
  b) "Instead of white rice, eat wild rice (which actually isn't rice)
  c) "Instead of coconut water, drink **Hint Water**

- "Drink lots of regular filtered water during the detox."
- I usually choose berries, green apples or pears as my fruit. If I eat other fruits, they are an occasional treat. When peaches come into season, I buy organic once and enjoy the treat, but then the craving is quelled, and I go back to the low sugar fruits above.
- One of the desserts that we serve company is fresh organic berries with coconut whipped cream. Yummy and low in sugar. High in good fats. Win Win!

Get off the sugar. Trust me. It's worth it and your body will thank you.

Additional reading

https://www.nytimes.com/2016/09/13/well/eat/how-the-sugar-industry-shifted-blame-to-fat.html?_r=0http://www.greenmedinfo.com/blog/22-ways-drinking-soda-will-shorten-your-life

http://www.dailymail.co.uk/home/you/article-2532775/Food-Sarah-Wilsons-I-Quit-Sugar.html

http://www.forbes.com/sites/alicegwalton/2012/08/30/how-much-sugar-are-americans-eating-infographic/#5ee4c6511f71

http://www.wellandgood.com/good-advice/addicted-to-sugar-sarah-wilson/

http://mamaglow.com/5-strategies-break-stealthy-sugar-addiction/

http://www.prevention.com/food/healthy-eating-tips/10-hidden-sugar-bombs/slide/10

http://www.bbcgoodfood.com/howto/guide/truth-about-sugar

http://articles.mercola.com/sites/articles/archive/2009/10/13/artificial-sweeteners-more-dangerous-than-you-ever-imagined.aspx

http://www.fitday.com/fitness-articles/nutrition/healthy-eating/top-number-most-dangerous-artificial-sweeteners.html

http://health.howstuffworks.com/wellness/food-nutrition/facts/artificial-sweetners-unhealthy-eco.htm

http://www.nytimes.com/interactive/2016/12/30/opinion/sunday/how-much-sugar-can-you-avoid-today.html

Recommended additional reading

The Blood Sugar Solution: The Ultra Healthy Program for Losing Weight, Preventing Disease, and Feeling Great Now! *Mark Hyman MD* (2014) from Little, Brown and Company

The Blood Sugar Solution 10-Day Detox Diet: Activate Your Body's Natural Ability to Burn Fat and Lose Weight Fast (2014) from Little, Brown and Company

I Quit Sugar: Your Complete 8-Week Detox Program and Cookbook Sarah Wilson Clarkson Potter Publishers (April 8, 2014)

JJ Virgin's Sugar Impact Diet: Drop 7 Hidden Sugars, Lose Up to 10 Pounds in Just 2 Weeks JJ Virgin Grand Central Life & Style; 1 edition (November 4, 2014)

Chapter 9

The perils of drinking soda

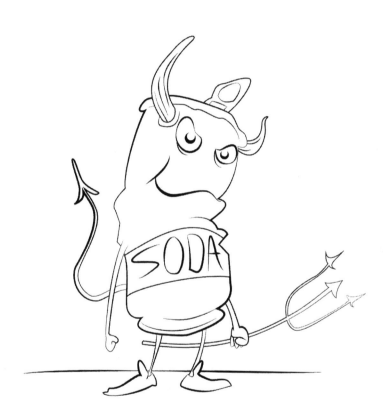

Dousing the flame of inflammation:

THE BIG TAKEAWAYS ON SODA

- Whether it is the one loaded with sugar or the one sweetened with artificial sweeteners, it is addictive and toxic to the body.
- Drinking soda causes the body inflammation.
- Drinking soda causes Metabolic Syndrome
- There is no value in soda for the body, none, no nutrients at all, but it is loaded with chemicals and causes the body incredible harm.
- Drink filtered water, which your body needs to thrive, instead. Add berries to it in the fridge and let the fruit infuse the water. Or drink Hint Water, instead of soda.

Our bodies need water. Most of us don't drink enough water. Sodas are often consumed in place of water.

There is no doubt that sugar tastes good. It has been shown to be addictive. And friends that I have that drink either sugar soda or diet soda would rather have their right arm cut off than give it up. But there is no denying, it is not good for you in any amount.

It doesn't matter whether it is soda with sugar, or diet soda or any of the products in-between. Soda is toxic, and you should not drink it, and certainly you should not let your children drink it.

If you have inflammation, it is not worth what it does to your body when you drink it.

Frankly, even if you don't have health issues, it is not ok for you to drinking coke or other carbonated sodas.

Drinking soda, either the sugary type or the fake sugar type, gives your body no nutrients, no benefit, and as determined in my chapter on Sugar (Part 3, Chapter 8), whether you are drinking a bottle full of real sugar, or a drink full of chemicals, your body suffers. Both are very harmful.

Just stop drinking soda, your health will thank you! It is not good for you in any quantity.

If you drink just two sodas a day, you increase your chance of having a heart attack by 40%.[195] You also increase your chance of dying from heart disease by 50%.

1 in 5 people drink a diet soda every day; that's 17% of the entire population or more than 5 million people. We haven't even added in the statistics of drinking soda with sugar, which has its own terrible effects on the body and on inflammation.[196] (See my chapter on sugar, Part 3, Chapter 8.)

Americans do not drink enough water, but instead, they drink 57 gallons of soda a year. Yikes![197]

In an article in **Medical Daily** by Samantha Olsen, January 22, 2015, titled *Soft Drink Dangers: 8 Ways Soda Negatively Affects Your Health* she states:

"As soon as soda is swallowed, the pancreas is notified and rapidly begins to create insulin in response to the sugar. Insulin is a hormone the body uses to move sugar from food or drink into the bloodstream, where cells are then able to use sugar for energy. Within just 20 minutes, blood sugar levels spike and the liver responds to the insulin by turning sugar into fat for storage.

Within 45 minutes of gulping down a single 20-ounce glass of soda, caffeine from the drink is fully absorbed, and as a result, your pupils dilate and blood pressure rises. The body produces more dopamine, which stimulates the pleasure centers of the brain — just like a low-grade line of cocaine.

When the hour chimes, the body begins to experience a blood sugar crash, which is around the same time a person reaches for their second soda, or for another sweet and sugar snack to suffice. Soda's connection to the obesity epidemic is so intertwined that Harvard researchers[198] " … have calculated that each additional soda consumed increases the risk of obesity 1.6 times."[199]

As an example, "Coke is a weak solution of cocaine with preservatives, colorants, and stabilizers, etc. This is legalized cocaine addiction plus pure poison. Diet Coke is even worse, because the aspartame in it replaces sugar, becoming pure neurotoxic poison."[200]

Also, these are the many health detriments

1. Sodas increase diabetes risk

2. They cause obesity

3. They are harmful to kidneys

4. They are harmful to the liver, which can't process all of the sugar or chemicals and stores the excess as fat causing fatty liver

5. Sodas have a lot of caffeine which is hard on the adrenals and dehydrates the body

6. Caffeine in coke blocks magnesium. We are becoming increasingly deficient in magnesium as a population. Magnesium is essential for more than 325 enzyme reactions in the body. Magnesium also plays a role in your body's detoxification processes and therefore is important for minimizing damage from environmental chemicals, heavy metals, and other toxins.

7. Carmel coloring is linked to vascular disease and linked to cancer[201]

8. Regular coke has 16 teaspoons of sugar in a 20 ounce can. How many people drink more than 1?[202]

9. Artificial sweeteners in diet coke interfere with the gut, cause leaky gut, and are linked to cancer. They are toxic substances. (See my Chapter 8 on sugar.) In diet sodas, aspartame is used as a substitute for sugar and can be more harmful. Diet sodas also increase the risk of metabolic syndrome, which causes belly fat, high blood sugar and raised cholesterol.

10. Soda cans are lined with BPA. (see my Chapter 10 on canned goods) BPA contains substances that are hormone disrupters.

11. Coke is a leading cause of osteoporosis because it leaches calcium from our bones.[203]

12. It is loaded with fructose (see my Chapter 8 on sugar)

13. It increases hunger since it shuts off your ability to realize satiation. (see Chapter 8 on Sugar)

14. There are no nutrients in a soda[204]

15. Soda PH runs between 2.5 and 3.9. This is very acidic and will dissolve tooth enamel.[205]

This is a list of things that coke is good for:[206]

1. It can clean the blood stains from your clothes.

2. You can soak pennies in Coke to polish them.

3. You can also use it to descale a kettle.

4. You can use it to clean the toilet. Just pour it in the toilet bowl, leave it a while, and then flush clean.

5. It can eliminate the grease stains from your clothes and fabrics.

6. You should pour some on the floor, and then hose off, to clean the oil stains in the garage.

7. Due to the high concentration of acids, it can kill slugs and snails.

8. Coke can help you eliminate the rust stains from your pool. You pour 2 liters of Coke into the pool and let it act for a while.

9. In Vietnam, my husband told me that soldiers cleaned the rust from their rifles using coke. (It also removed the bluing).

10. To clean car battery terminals pour a little coke on the contacts and let it sit a moment.

11. To remove gum stuck in hair, dip it in a bit of Coke and keep it there for 2 minutes, and then wipe it off.

12. You can also use it to clean engines.

13. Coke can help you remove paint from your metal furniture. You should dip a towel in it, and apply it on the paint stains.

14. Pour a bit of Coke on the kitchen floor, leave it to act, and then wipe it to clean the tile grout.

15. Coke can help you fade or remove the hair dye.

16. Coke can efficiently polish Chrome.

17. Use it to clean the stains from vitreous china.

18. To clean the marker stains on the carpet, pour a bit of it on the spot, and then scrub, and rinse with soapy water.

19. You should pour some Coke in your burnt pans, leave it to act, and rinse the pan to clean it.

I think you get the point. If you want to stop your pain, stop your inflammation, and return to wellness, **NEVER** drink soda again.

Drink water. Your body really, really needs water. You can add lemon or a few small pieces of fresh berries or fruit to your water and enjoy it that way instead. One drop of Stevia makes it sweet. Your body will thank you. And it's another important step to your return to wellness.

Chapter 10

Canned Goods

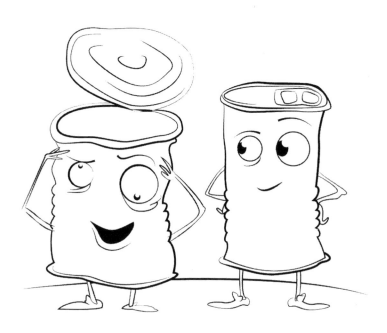

Dousing the flame of inflammation:

THE BIG TAKEAWAYS ON CANNED GOODS

- Most cans have a BPA lining with is believed to be an endocrine disruptor in the body.
- There is "evidence of absence" as to whether or not BPA causes other health issues. Even though there are no independent studies available, there are issues showing up with animals.
- Canned goods are not regulated, so even if BPA is not used, companies are reluctant to declare that, because there is no law about how much trace BPA is allowed and they don't want to be caught with trace amounts.
- You can check the EWG site for the amounts of toxins in the canned goods you are purchasing.
- SPROUTS own brand is BPA free. There are charts on the EWG site under FOOD SCORES that show which brands are and which are not a potential problem.
- If something you love is on the list of items with BPA list, call them. I use Rao Spaghetti Sauce; they were on the BPA list, so I called them. They responded that the BPA is under a seal on the lid and that there is no leakage of BPA into their product. There is no way to know if that is true, but I will continue using their sauce. You decide what you want to do.
- Do the best you can to avoid toxins. Whatever you do is better than if you were not avoiding any of them.

You are probably aware that there is a concern about BPA linings in cans, especially for pregnant mothers, but also, to some extent for the rest of us.

"The lining of most cans contain BPA, which has been linked to heart disease, diabetes, poor memory, reproductive disorders, and more. This toxic chemical is infused into the food stored inside the can."[208]

BPA is a synthetic estrogen in the lining of our canned goods. It is unregulated. Although many companies have committed to getting rid of the BPA lining, in many cases there is no plan to do so. Even some companies committed to removing the BPA think they have solved the issue with their suppliers, only to discover that there is still BPA in the cans that they are using.

It is further complicated by the fact that companies that are BPA free don't want to put it on their products since it is unregulated, and not defined by law what BPA levels should be. So, if there are trace elements in their cans, they don't want to be caught short.

EWG writes in **BPA in Canned Food: Health hazards of BPA**, June 3, 2015:

"Bisphenol A has been shown to mimic thyroid and sex hormones in people and animals. It has been associated with a wide variety of health problems, including altered brain and nervous system development and changes in the reproductive system. Much of the evidence of BPA toxicity is based on laboratory animal studies, where low exposures to BPA during pregnancy or early life can permanently affect fertility, behavior and body size and can predispose animals to later life cancers (Vandenberg 2013)."

"There is less than definitive evidence of BPA toxicity to people, but observational studies associates BPA exposure with a host of issues, including behavioral changes in children and diseases like obesity and heart disease."[209]

EWG is especially concerned about pregnant woman and small children. Children cannot detoxify the chemicals as readily as adults and then the chemicals cause problems.

EWG makes the following recommendations:

"Substitute fresh, frozen, or dried food for canned.

"Purchase food in alternative packaging, such as glass.

"For those who cannot avoid BPA epoxy can linings, rinsing canned beans, fruit, and vegetables in water may help lower the level of BPA in the food.

"Never heat food in the can.

"Choose canned foods from **EWG's** *Best Players* or *Better Players* lists of brands and companies that attest to using BPA-free linings in all or some of their canned products. Search *EWG's Food Scores* for specific products."[210]

There are two charts on the EWG site, one for companies that use BPA and another that has can goods that are BPA free. It is worth taking a look, especially if you are pregnant or have small children, but also since I am writing this book for people struggling with inflammation, this is a chemical that is best avoided.

You can find the charts on the EWG site under http://www.ewg.org/research/bpa-canned-food.

Sprouts Farmers Markets is listed as BPA free for their branded canned goods. But Whole Foods is not on either chart. These Whole Foods products may or may not have BPA. Look for the words no BPA on the can. I did recently see it on Whole Foods some of their own canned goods under the **365** label.

Chapter 11

Soy

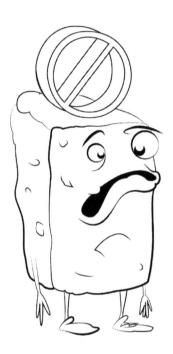

Dousing the flame of inflammation:

THE BIG TAKEAWAYS ON SOY

- Avoid GMO Soy. It appears that the pesticides used to grow GMO soy cause disease.
- Eat fermented soy; they are good for you.
- Avoid soy infant formulas.

Soy is on my sensitivity list. I do miss soy sauce, but when cooking at home, Coconut Aminos are a great substitute. When out, where I have no control, I avoid it. My reaction to anything with soy is instant, and painful.

Is Soy Good or Bad For You?

I decided to let the experts talk for themselves.

The head nutritionist from the Cleveland Clinic, Kristen Kirkpatrick, said on the Dr. Oz Show[212], that soy is good for us. It is a complete protein; it is high in fiber, high in Potassium and Magnesium, Manganese, Selenium, Copper, Phosphorus, Iron, Calcium, Vitamin B6, Folate, Riboflavin (B2), Thiamin (B1) and Vitamin K. It reduces cardiovascular disease, and it reduces breast cancer risks.

The best soy is fermented, tempeh, miso (high in B-12) and natto, which is very popular in Japan. Also, soy sauce if it is fermented in the traditional way.

The high isoflavones in soy are plant estrogen, so she states that it is less potent than it is usually portrayed to be.

An article in Scientific American,[213] *Could Eating Too Much Soy Be Bad For You?* By Lindsey Konkel 11/01/2009 disagrees with this, and she stated that new studies show that these plant estrogens do interfere with reproduction in mice and that most likely they interfere with reproduction in humans. Although not proven, these scientists have a particular concern with infant formulas and the long-term risks to the child.

"There is significant evidence that soy-based infant formula can cause harm, both via its isoflavone content and via its unnaturally high content of manganese and aluminum." Soy is an interesting food to me. I have never enjoyed it, and it ends up it is high on my sensitivity list, so it's just as well that I only ate it on occasion.

In an article from Authority Nutrition[214], *Is Soy Bad For You, or Good? The Shocking Truth,* they state "The respectable number of nutrients listed above needs to be taken with a grain of salt because soybeans are also very high in **phytates**, substances that bind minerals and reduce their absorption." In other words, in spite of all of the juicy minerals in soy, the body doesn't get to enjoy them because they are chelated out. They also point out that the oil in soybeans is Omega-6, which should be limited in our diets. We get more than we need in everyday eating.

This article does see this benefit to soy – "There is some evidence that soy can lower cholesterol levels, although studies show conflicting results. Men who consume soy are at a lower risk of developing prostate cancer in old age."

There is an article in the New York Times, today: **This Pesticide Is Prohibited in Britain. Why Is It Still Being Exported?** 12/20/2016 about another pesticide that is banned in Europe, but used abundantly on Soy crops in the US called Paraquet.[215] The article states that studies have shown a direct correlation between eating Paraquet on crops (which are soy crops) and Parkinson's. If you are going to eat soy, make sure it is organic.

In an article in the Huffington Post, by Dr. Joseph Mercola, **The Health Dangers Of Soy** 8/23/2013 he brings up the fact that soy is 90% GMO, a big negative, and it is grown with Glyphosate. (See my Chapter 6 on GMO's.) Other strong negatives on soy are:[216]

1. "High Phytic Acid (Phytates): Reduces assimilation of calcium, magnesium, copper, iron and zinc. Phytic acid in soy is not neutralized by ordinary preparation methods such as soaking, sprouting, and long, slow cooking, but only with long fermentation. High-phytate diets have caused growth problems in children.

2. "Trypsin inhibitors: Interferes with protein digestion and may cause pancreatic disorders. In test animals, trypsin inhibitors in soy caused stunted growth.

3. "Goitrogens: Potent agents that block your synthesis of thyroid hormones and can cause hypothyroidism and thyroid cancer. In infants, consumption of soy formula has been linked to autoimmune thyroid disease. Goitrogens interfere with iodine metabolism.

4. "Phytoestrogens/Isoflavones: Plant compounds resembling human estrogen can block your normal estrogen and disrupt endocrine function, cause infertility, and increase your risk for breast cancer.

5. "Hemagglutinin: A clot-promoting substance that causes your red blood cells to clump, making them unable to absorb and distribute oxygen to your tissues.

6. "Synthetic Vitamin D: Soy foods increase your body's vitamin D requirement, which is why companies add synthetic vitamin D-2 to soymilk (a toxic form of vitamin D).

7. "Vitamin B-12: Soy contains a compound resembling vitamin B-12 that cannot be used by your body, so soy foods can contribute to B-12 deficiency, especially among vegans.

8. "Protein Denaturing: Fragile proteins are denatured during high temperature processing to make soy protein isolate and textured vegetable protein (TVP). Chemical processing of soy protein results in the formation of toxic lysinoalanine and highly carcinogenic nitrosamines.

9. "MSG: Free glutamic acid, or MSG, is a potent neurotoxin. MSG is formed during soy food processing; plus, additional MSG is often added to mask soy's unpleasant taste. (Health Muse note: This is a biggie; MSG is really bad for you)

10. "Aluminum and Manganese: Soy foods contain high levels of aluminum, which is toxic to your nervous system and kidneys, and manganese, which wreaks havoc on your baby's immature metabolic system."

Wellness Mama in her article *Is Soy Healthy* January 4, 2016, agrees with Dr. Mercola.

Latest research from my newsletter, ***The Wellness Blaylock Report***, January 2017 from Dr. Randall Blaylock, genetically modified soy can cause sterility. Yikes[217]

They all agree that fermented soy is good for you.

So, in conclusion, if I could eat soy, I would restrict it to fermented soy; this includes tempeh, miso, and natto, which is very popular in Japan. Also, soy sauce if it is fermented in the traditional way. I would try to buy all of these fermented soy foods in an organic version.

I would avoid using soy in infant formulas as there does seem to be a bit of a risk there, which appears to be agreed upon.

Chapter 12

Dairy

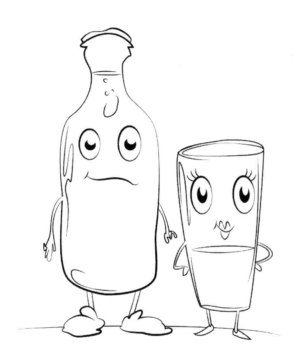

Dousing the flame of inflammation:

THE BIG TAKEAWAYS ON DAIRY

- Only use full fat dairy.
- Only buy organic dairy products from grass-fed cows to avoid synthetic growth hormones, antibiotics and the stress hormones from factory farmed meat.
- Raw milk is a good choice for additional nutrients and better taste.
- Yogurt is good for you, but only buy full fat with no added sugar.
- If you eat cheese, if it is cow cheese, make sure it is organic, or eat sheep or goat cheese. Watch the salt content on the label.

Dairy was the first category that I discovered I was highly sensitive to when I started my journey five years ago. Probably my most favorite thing in the world is cheese, and I don't get to eat it anymore. When I fall off the wagon and eat cheese, hoping that the cheese won't cause inflammation, bingo, I get a flare, so it's just not worth trying anymore. It doesn't matter if it is a cow, sheep or goat, I can't eat dairy.

It is a common thing for people to be sensitive to, so I am not alone.

The good news is that I can eat ghee, which is clarified butter. Clarified means the milk proteins have been removed, and these proteins are what my body can no longer tolerate; I am sensitive to the whey and casein protein in the milk. Ghee is just as tasty as butter to me, so it solves a multitude of sins in eliminating dairy.

But the bigger question is, is dairy good for anyone? This is what I found:

75% of the world is lactose intolerant.[219] The primary carbohydrate in dairy is lactose, a "milk sugar" that is made of the two simple sugars glucose and galactose. North America, Europe, and Australia, don't have this intolerance as much as the rest of the world.

Whole milk from grass fed cows is quite nutritious. If it is organic grass fed cow milk, it also has avoided most of the hormones, antibiotics and pesticides/herbicides that are in factory cow milk.[220] Grass fed cow dairy has omega three fatty acids which we need[221], and it has fat soluble vitamins like K-2 that are essential to human bones. I am talking about milk only in this regard, not cheese, which we will get to in a second.

The most nutritious milk is whole raw milk from grass fed cows. It is not as risky as once thought and has many benefits over conventional pasteurized milk.[222]

Low-fat or nonfat dairy, however, is not healthy and has had the fat replaced with dry milk (which has its own health hazards).

Full-fat grass-fed dairy can reduce the risks of diabetes II.[223] This is not true of low-fat or nonfat dairy. Full-fat grass-fed dairy is also linked to reduced obesity.[224] [225]

If the milk is from grass-fed cows, it is also linked to reduced heart disease[226] and reduced strokes[227]. A study in Australia showed a 69% drop in heart disease if grass-fed organic milk was regularly drunk.

Fermented dairy products like yogurt and kefir may be even better if they are made from grass-fed milk. They contain probiotic bacteria that can have numerous health benefits

Factory farmed cows are given growth hormones and antibiotics to reduce infection and those substances remain in the milk. These drugs are harmful to the human body.

Factory farmed milk often has contaminants in it.

There are new studies that show the calcium in milk is different from human milk, and we can't absorb it. New studies have shown that drinking milk can reduce calcium in our bones.[228] Statistics show, in countries where less milk is drunk, there is less osteoporosis. "And the 12 years long Harvard Nurses' Health Study found that those who consumed the most calcium from dairy foods broke more bones than those who rarely drank milk. The Harvard Nurses' Health Study is a broad study based on 77,761 women aged 34 to 59 years of age.[229]"

Milk is an acidifying protein, so the body sacrifices the bones by pulling out the calcium in the bones by neutralizing the acid to save the kidneys. Pasteurization increases the acid level.[230]

Growth hormone or rBGH, in conventional factory milk causes several cancers, especially breast cancer, and makes the cancers more aggressive. (Another fantastic **Monsanto** product, aarrggh!)[231]

rBGH is banned in the EU.

The Monsanto rBGH/BST Milk Wars Handbook Dr. Samuel Epstein[232]

- "rBGH makes cows sick. Monsanto has been forced to admit to about 20 veterinary health risks on its Posilac label including mastitis and udder inflammation
- "rBGH milk is contaminated by pus from mastitis induced by rBGH, and antibiotics used to treat the mastitis.
- "rBGH milk is contaminated by the GE hormone which can be absorbed through the gut and induce immunological effects.
- "rBGH milk is chemically and nutritionally very different from natural milk.
- "rBGH milk is supercharged with high levels of a natural growth factor (IGF-1), excess levels of which have been incriminated as major causes of breast, colon, and prostate cancers.
- "rBGH factory farms pose a major threat to the viability of small dairy farms. Thus, rBGH enriches Monsanto while posing risks, but no benefits to the entire U.S. population."

Milk is considered a mucus-producing food and is clinically thought to aggravate congestion."[233] *Is Milk Good For You,* an article in **How Stuff Works** states: "Johns Hopkins physician, Dr. Frank Oski, has even written a book that shares his experiences of decreased rates of strep throat infection once children removed milk from their diets. Often, these conditions resolve or improve when milk is removed or eliminated from the diet." Conditions at factory farmed dairies are horrific. The stress hormones from a factory farmed cow pass into the milk and you.

In addition:

1. Conventional cows are fed GMO feed, raised in unhealthy situations, so they have to get large amounts of antibiotics to keep them healthy,

2. Confined cows have virtually no Vitamin D, so a synthetic Vitamin D is added to the milk. What we get from the sun is D-3. What the cow gets is synthesized D-2, and it's not remotely the same.

Organic yogurt that does not have hormones added to it is quite good for you. (Call the dairy of the brand you buy to make sure.) Make sure that it has no added sugar (most yogurts are loaded with sugar, remember 4 grams equals one teaspoon, so read the label)

So, let's talk about skim (nonfat) milk and low-fat milk.

They are not healthy. Do NOT drink them.

1. They were created to make dairies money. By skimming off the cream, the dairy keeps the most expensive part of the milk and sells you the balance.

2. Skim milk has an unappealing taste and color, so powdered milk products are added back into the milk for color and flavor. "What's so bad about powdered milk? Well, in the manufacturing process, liquid milk is forced through tiny holes at very high pressure, which causes the cholesterol in the milk to oxidize, and causes toxic nitrates to form. Oxidized cholesterol contributes to the buildup of plaque in the arteries, while unoxidized cholesterol from unprocessed foods is actually an antioxidant to help fight inflammation in the body. The proteins found in powdered milk are so denatured that they are unrecognizable by the body and contribute to inflammation."[234] Furthermore, dairies are not required to list powdered milk on the ingredients, because the government still considers it "milk."

3. An article by Aviva Romm in **Living Traditionally** called *6 Secrets you Don't Know About Skim Milk*, April 14, 2014,[235] states "Also legal, are the injections of recombinant bovine growth hormones, or rBGH, a **known carcinogen** banned in virtually every industrialized nation in the world, except the United States. The 'recombinant' part of the growth hormone

means that it was **genetically modified** from the cow's natural growth hormones to stimulate increased milk production."

4. There is very little nutritional value to nonfat and low-fat milk. All of the nutrients have been removed.

5. Skim milk and 1% milk are associated with weight gain. If you are not eating fat, you are consistently hungry.

6. There is no need to eliminate the fat from the milk. There are no health benefits, and there are detriments as noted above.[236]

Finally, dairy is not essential for good health, for your children or you.

Ok, now let's talk about cheese.

- Cheese is a source of CLA, conjugated linoleic acid, which is good for you
- Cheese may reduce tooth decay
- There are studies that show that cheese reduces cancer risk, and there are studies that show cheese increases cancer risk. This one is a draw. Studies prove both.
- Whether or not it increases heart disease is also a draw. Studies show both.
- Watch the amount of salt on the labeling. Some cheeses have much more than others
- Cheese is Americans largest source of saturated fat. It should only be eaten in moderation at best.
- There are growth hormones and antibiotics in the cheese, just like in our milk. See above. Buy cheese that is organic from grass fed cows. All sheep eat grass, so this would not be the case with sheep's cheese. Goats are not factory farmed, so they have been eating their natural diet.
- Cheese happens to be especially addictive because of an ingredient called casein, a protein found in all milk products. During digestion, casein releases opiates called casomorphins.

In an October 22, 2016, article from the **Los Angeles Times,** *Cheese Is Really Crack; Study Reveals Cheese is as Addictive as Drugs* [237] by Jenna Harris, states "[Casomorphins] really play with the dopamine receptors and trigger that addictive element," registered dietitian Cameron Wells.

"Leading the charge against cheese is Dr. Neal Barnard MD, founder, and president of the **Physicians Committee for Responsible Medicine.** He's the kind of guy who calls cheese 'dairy crack.' If that sounds a tad dramatic, consider what happens in your body when you digest cheese, a process Dr. Barnard explained in his book, **21-Day Weight Loss Kickstart,** Grand Central Life & Style; 3rd edition (February 28, 2011) and summarized in an email."[238]

No wonder I still miss my cheese. I was addicted to it, like crack. Geeze!!!

Studies are inconclusive as to whether dairy and cheese are good or bad for us. How does your body feel when you drink milk or eat cheese?

It is clear that nonfat and low-fat, however, are bad.

So, if you decide to avoid dairy, what do you use instead? I drink almond milk (I buy **Califia Farms**.) Make sure you buy one that is unsweetened, and that doesn't have carrageenan in it. Remember to read all of the ingredients, and if you can't pronounce them, it's the wrong product. I also buy almond yogurt from Kite Hill (Whole Foods) and Almond Ricotta from Kite Hill. They also make some soft cheeses, but they are not my thing.

Alternatives to dairy milk:

- Coconut milk
- Cashew milk. Easy to make, just be sure to soak the organic cashews overnight. No need to strain. Forager also makes a yummy cashew milk available at Whole Foods.
- I recently tried Pea milk, it was pretty good.

Chapter 13

Sensitivities

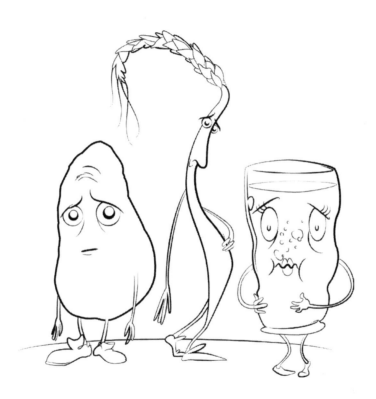

Dousing the flame of inflammation:

THE BIG TAKEAWAYS ON SENSITIVITIES

- Discovering your sensitivities is critical to heal from inflammation
- There are two approaches, the Elimination Diet, and/or taking Cyrex Sensitivity tests.
- My sensitivities were a combination of the most usual suspects and things found on the sensitivity tests I took.
- Learn to listen to your body. It will start to tell you when something you are eating is causing a reaction.
- Gluten sensitivities are broken into two groups, Celiac, and non-Celiac. Both cause horrific inflammation. If you suspect you have a gluten issue, find a practitioner that specializes in this area. Conventional doctors often think gluten sensitivity is a fad. (My original conventional doctor did.)
- Once you know your sensitivities, adjust your diet to eliminate them.
- Avoiding sensitivities is a huge step towards reducing inflammation.

As discussed in my Chapter 4 on autoimmunity, to heal the gut it is important to identify the food items that you are sensitive to and eliminate them. Eliminating the foods that you are sensitive to is critical. Then, you need to start eating real food and eliminating the fake foods. These two changes had a huge impact on reducing my pain. Once I stopped eating foods that I was sensitive to, my body responded in about two weeks, and the pain started to fade away. It didn't completely make my pain go away, but it certainly improved how I felt, and I was able to sleep again without lying in bed with pain. Finally, I could get out of bed in the morning and function, because these foods we no longer in my diet.

As I mentioned earlier, I had had "allergy" tests with my conventional MD, and all I was allergic to was the adhesive tape that held the test on my back. An allergy is different than a sensitivity.

The reaction to an allergy is immediate, and severe, like an allergy to peanuts or an allergy to shellfish.

"True food allergies are based on exposure to a specific protein component of a food. The immune system incorrectly perceives the protein as a threat and produces antibodies in response. With repeated exposure, cells release histamine and other biochemicals in response to the allergenic food. It is these chemicals that cause the allergy symptoms."[240]

"Food allergies have an immune basis, so you experience symptoms every time you consume a food. Typical symptoms include skin rash and swelling and hives, often in the throat; severe **reactions can be life-threatening**."[241] In observing friends with food allergies, there seems to be a much faster reaction time to the problem food. People seem to react more severely each time there is contact with the allergen.

Robyn O'Brien clarifies the difference between allergies and sensitivities, in her article called *Food Allergies & Food Sensitivities: Know the Difference* from her website from March 15, 2015, She is a food advocate that got involved defending her children's health. "Both allergies and sensitivities have the same ultimate cause: the immune system's overreaction to apparently harmless food. According to internationally acclaimed author and physician Kenneth Bock, M.D., there's also quite a bit of overlap between IgE and IgG (see information below) symptoms. Both can contribute to inflammatory responses in multiple body systems."[242]

The difference is timing; allergies create an immediate response. Sensitivities create a slower response in the body but are still a key factor that leads to leaky gut, inflammation, and pain in the body. Like allergies, food sensitivities start to destroy tissues in the body and attack brain tissue, joints, skin and organ systems.

Conventional medicine overlooks the role of food sensitivities in the body. (Which is one reason our current health care model is failing and as a result, autoimmune is rapidly on the rise.)

Sensitivities are a significant cause of pain. If they are not removed, the gut cannot heal, and the inflammation continues. With the inflammation, comes the pain.

"This is imperative to improve your quality of life and reduce the risk of chronic degenerative disease. Additionally, the individual notices improved energy, sleep, brain function, physical appearance and mood. They also have less pain, less acne/eczema, less fatigue and improved metabolism, lean body tissue development, and fat loss."[243]

"Are we allergic to food, or are we increasingly allergic to what has been done to it?"

ROBYN O'BRIEN **FOOD MATTERS**

The same can be said of sensitivities.

My conventional doctor never suggested that we test for sensitivities. And, as it ended up, this test was a big part of the keys of the kingdom to my health.

There are two approaches to sensitivity by the functional medicine community.

The first is a lower cost option, and that is to remove foods that are known to create inflammation and sensitivity; wait several months, and then start to introduce them back in, one at a time, and see how your body reacts. This process is called a Food Elimination Test.

I did a version of this when I just got started with my first functional Chiropractor and Nutritionist. He did test for dairy and gluten sensitivities and then stopped me from eating the other most common problematic foods.

So, right off the bat, we removed gluten, and dairy, and beans, corn, nightshades and soy. We also changed the oils I could use and limited them to the oils I use today, ghee, coconut, avocado, and California olive oil*, which are all healthy choices. Other oils are often the culprit that causes inflammation.

When I got the gluten and dairy tests for sensitivity back, I was indeed, sensitive to these foods. But my problem was far from solved.

I never liked soy, so it was ok with me that I needed to eliminate soy from my diet. I had a strong reaction to casein and whey, proteins in dairy, so goodbye milk and cheese. (I dearly love cheese, and have tried to reintroduce it a couple of times, but my body gains 5 pounds over night, I swell up and get pain, so I have become resolved to the fact that cheese is gone.) *frown*

After six months, I reintroduced gluten and didn't react, but since I was now actively involved in getting well, I understood that gluten was a protein that my body couldn't digest well, so I only eat it on occasion. It too can be a cause of inflammation. We will discuss gluten further below.

However, I still had a lot of inflammation, and this is where sensitivity tests come in.

My functional MD ordered a complete profile of tests from **Cyrex** to find my sensitivities. Had we not tested, I would never have known that these were the items to avoid. The elimination diet would have never found them. We ordered the Celiac and Gluten Sensitivity test, an IgG test and an IgG spice profile, an IgE inhalant profile, an IgM mold profile and a Veg add on. These tests are not inexpensive, but if you do them all at once, you know what to avoid to stop the pain. We are talking about pain, and you are totally worth knowing what needs to be avoided, no matter what the cost.

There is a new sensitivity test available for home use. It is from a company called **Everly Well**. You can get a battery of tests done for $199. At least, this is a start to see what your problem foods are.

What a sensitivity test is looking for:

Dr. Jocker's explains on his website in an article called **Food *Sensitivity Testing* Major Immune Factors:**[244]

Dr. David Jockers, a functional nutritionist, states: "Think of these guys like the branches of the military. We have the Army, Navy, Marines, Coast Guard, etc. Within these branches, we have additional arms such as the Navy Seals. The immune system is set up similar in that it has different branches and arms. The three major ones associated with food allergies and sensitivities are IgE, IgG, and IgA.

"**IgE or immunoglobulin E** allergies are immediate responses to a foreign substance that has entered the body. These foreign substances can come from food or breathing in different chemicals, pollen, dust, cat hair, etc. IgE allergies can cause very serious symptoms like difficulty breathing, swelling, and hives. In even more serious cases IgE reactions can lead to anaphylactic shock.

"**IgG or Immunoglobulin G** are antibodies that provide long-term resistance to infections. They have a much longer half-life than the traditional IgE allergy. This is where food sensitivities come in because they are much subtler and most people live with them for years, if not their entire lives.

"IgA or Immunoglobulin A are antibodies that are part of our body's natural immune defense within the mucosal membrane. These antibodies are in the saliva, digestive tract, sinuses, etc. When there is inflammatory activity in the gut (which is very common), there, is quite often elevated IgA antibodies.

"Those who understand mucosal immunology know that when the body is exposed to an antigen through the digestive tract, the body will produce IgA based antibodies first. This happens before IgG, IgE or IgM.

"Some of the antibodies from the salivary glands are also secreted into the blood. So, IgA can be detected first in saliva and then in blood. If the patient consumes more and more of the same antigen, an inflammatory reaction may occur in the gut, causing the tight junctions to open. Antigens flood into the submucosa; from there they migrate into the regional lymph nodes and then into the circulation. At this point, the body will begin producing IgM or IgG antibodies against those food antigens."

Below, is my list of my sensitivities? If I had only done an elimination test, I would not have found most of these problem foods and spices. It took the sensitivity test to find them.

- Corn
- Dairy (butter, cheese, milk)
- Fennel
- Sage
- Basil
- Mustard
- Soy
- Mint
- Green beans
- Artichokes
- Canola oil
- Chicken
- Flax

- Potatoes
- Buckwheat
- Olive trees
- June Grass
- Cat dander (I do have cats, and in spite of the testing I seem to be ok) (in other words, I am not giving them up. Ha!)
- Pityroporum obiculare mold

We were eating artichokes once a week. Who knew that they were creating antigens that were attacking my body?

Sensitivity could take a couple of days for the body to react, and it can impact your body for a couple of weeks.

My body is ultra-sensitive. I react within a couple of hours, and if I take extra curcumin bp, quercetin and resveratrol, (all antioxidants) I can, reduce the inflammation in maybe three days.

I still avoid things with gluten, which are wheat (under many different names), barley, and rye. So, not eating those items, and staying away from flax, buckwheat, and potatoes becomes problematic since many foods that are eliminated for gluten are made with one of those five foods in them. (Bread, protein shakes, crackers, cookies.) Even most commercial gluten-free items use something on my list. (And these products often have other questionable ingredients.) Ok, I have learned to cook my own food around it. (A lot of gluten free foods have junk in them. One of the ingredients I see most often is cellulose which is tree pulp. I have found great recipes and also some great breads that are gluten free and healthy. Check my website under resources for more information.)

And it's worth it. I can't begin to tell you how much better I feel avoiding these items. Every once in a while, I accidentally get a food with one of these ingredients in it, probably at a restaurant, or sometimes as a guest in someone's home, no matter how careful I try to be, and inevitably, I have a "flare" and wake up in pain, all bloated and swollen and 5 pounds fatter. Yikes! It often takes a week to subside.

You may have sensitivities to foods other than mine; nuts are common, sometimes with gluten, sometimes as a stand-alone sensitivity. Corn and beans are also common. Nightshades are common.

Gluten is an entirely different issue and shows itself in many different ways causing inflammation and pain and disease. There is gluten in wheat, barley, and rye. These are also products that are often heavily sprayed with pesticides and herbicides. And the gluten molecule is a larger size than our gut can handle. We aren't born with enzymes to break down the gluten protein. In other words, gluten often causes leaky gut even where there is no sensitivity.

If the tests above have not resolved your issue, then complete testing for gluten becomes critical. And if you have gluten sensitivity, you must stay away from it, watch for cross-contamination, and be vigilant.

The leading expert on gluten, Dr. Tom O'Bryan states, in his blog called *The Conundrum of Gluten Sensitivity and Autoimmunity, Why the Tests are Often Wrong* from his website:

"We recognize the now well-known fact, that Gluten Sensitivity may manifest as Celiac Disease, or it may manifest outside of the intestines; one of the ways of expanding our diagnostic range is to focus on whether or not our immune system is saying that gluten is a problem. We may know where the problem is manifesting, or we may not. But if our immune system is saying "We've got a problem here," you should pay attention. As a comparison, if your car is running fine on the highway at 60 miles per hour, do you listen when the immune system of the car (the dashboard gauges) says "we've got a problem here", and the hot light has it up, or do we say "the cars running fine? I don't see or feel any problem," and keep driving? I think most would agree that is not a very wise move. The same is true for your body. You may 'feel' a problem; you may not. The point I want to make is that we will benefit from 'listening' to what our immune system is saying to us. We just have to be able to hear what it's trying to say."[245]

Gluten sensitivity includes Celiac Disease, which affects the intestines. But it is much bigger than that. "There is a new blood test, looking at 12 different peptides of gluten, not just Gliadin. This test is known as Array 3 from Cyrex Labs." Ask your doctor to run this test for you. It must be ordered by a physician. If they are hesitant, find a Certified Gluten Practitioner, and there is a link on Dr. O'Brien's website www.TheDr.com.

Dr. O'Bryan continues: "And my personal prayer is that as a result of this expanded test looking for a reaction to gluten, we no longer miss those with earlier stages of Celiac Disease and Gluten Sensitivity, thus being able to calm down the 'fire in the belly', the hot light on the dashboard, before the engine blows up. Before the diagnosis of Attention Deficit Hyperactivity Disorder, before the diagnosis of Autoimmune Thyroid Disease, before the diagnosis of Type I Diabetes, before the diagnosis of migraines, before the loss of pregnancy, ... And doctors will have the tools to truly guide their patients in increasing one's health. Tuning the engine before it blows up with a diagnosable disease. So, our bodies can carry us through life purring instead of rumbling along."

Dr. Josh Axe states in a blog on his website called *Gluten Intolerance Symptoms & Treatment Methods*:[246]

"Symptoms of gluten intolerance (or NCGS) nonceliac gluten sensitivity, are widespread and can include:

- "Digestive and IBS symptoms, including abdominal pain, cramping, bloating, constipation or diarrhea
- "'Brain fog', difficulty concentrating and trouble remembering information
- "Frequent headaches
- "Mood-related changes, including anxiety and increased depression symptoms
- "Ongoing low energy levels and chronic fatigue syndrome
- "Muscle and joint pains
- "Numbness and tingling in the arms and legs
- "Reproductive problems and infertility
- "Skin issues, including dermatitis, eczema, rosacea and skin rashes
- "Nutrient deficiencies, including anemia (iron deficiency)
- "Higher risk for learning disabilities, including autism and ADHD
- "Possibly a higher risk for neurological and psychiatric diseases, including Alzheimer's, dementia and schizophrenia.

- "Celiac disease symptoms typically include:
- "Bloating
- "Cramping and abdominal pain
- "Diarrhea or constipation
- "Trouble concentrating or "brain fog."
- "Changes in weight
- "Sleep disturbances including insomnia
- "Chronic fatigue or lethargy
- "Nutrient deficiencies (malnutrition) due to absorption problems within the digestive tract
- "Chronic headaches
- "Joint or bone pains
- "Changes in mood, such an anxiety
- "Tingling numbness in the hands and feet
- "Seizures
- "Irregular periods, infertility or recurrent miscarriage
- "Canker sores inside the mouth
- "Thinning hair and dull skin."

Finding a solution for these issues and Celiac or non-Celiac sensitivity to gluten can be very difficult to identify. For more information read Jennifer Esposito's book **Jennifer's Way: My Journey with Celiac Disease—What Doctors Don't Tell You and How You Can Learn to Live Again**. Da Capo Lifelong Books; Reprint edition (April 28, 2015) Jennifer was the actress on **Blue Bloods** that suddenly disappeared from the cast because of illness. Now with her gluten issues under control, she is a regular this season on **NCIS**. Her story will frighten and enlighten you.

If your doctor is hesitant to order the Cyrex tests, there are many functional practitioners with many different degrees that can. You can find functional practitioners by searching here. https://www.functionalmedicine.org/practitioner. A functional MD, a functional nurse practitioner, a functional Naturopath, a functional Chiropractor, can all get you the information that you need to remove your sensitivities from your diet.

As a health coach, I can help you navigate how to eliminate these foods, and how to eat so that you are not deprived. You can thrive around your sensitivities. There are yummy alternatives.

* The olive oil market has been corrupted by the mafia. They are watering down the olive oil exported from Europe and not listing the other ingredients. These are often oils that are bad for the body. California passed a law that all olive oils that come from California MUST be pure 100% olive oil. Buy Californian olive oil to save your health. Or, look for the International Olive Council seal to ensure it is pure. Only buy extra virgin, cold pressed.

Chapter 14

Factory farmed meat, chicken and fish and good alternatives

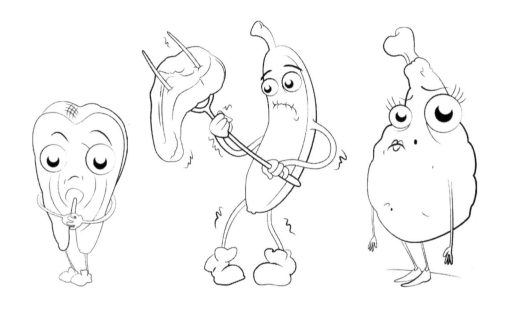

Dousing the flame of inflammation:

THE BIG TAKEAWAYS ON FACTORY FARMED MEATS AND FISH

- I will spare you the gruesome details about factory farming methods. It's difficult to read. It is disgusting. It is far worse than anything I could imagine and uglier than I have ever believed. The animals are raised under inhumane conditions. There is no care to how much pain the animal is put through, to increase its meat before it is butchered.
- If you want to become informed on these practices, articles are easy to find on the internet. You will try to avoid factory farmed meat for the rest of your life, once you read the facts.
- All stress hormones go into our food supply, which is not healthy for us.
- The use of growth hormones, antibiotics, and other chemicals is blatant on these animals. This practice creates complications for us, the consumer, because the antibiotics in the food affect our gut bacteria. The gut bacteria becomes resistant to the antibiotic. If we are required to take antibiotics for a serious health reason, the antibiotics will not work. (I had this problem at one point) We are creating an entire population of Super Bugs.
- There are some new regulations to control antibiotic use on animals[248] but these new regulations have tons of wiggle room, so real change is yet to be seen.
- Buy pastured organic meats, the same rules apply to organic meat as apply to organic veggies – they don't have the GMO component that is poisoning us.

DO NOT EAT FACTORY FARMED MEAT IF AT ALL POSSIBLE. Become Informed.

I attempt to eat Pagan.[249] This is a term coined by Mark Hyman, MD and it means that ¾ of your plate should be veggies and that the meat at that meal should be the size of your palm, and considered to be a condiment.

The health community is clearly confused as to whether we should eat meat or not. I follow a Functional Heart Doctor, Dr. Joel Kahn, who strongly recommends a Vegan diet.

Paleo followers strongly believe that there are things in meat that we need for optimal body performance.

I like the idea of Pagan because it is a compromise between the two schools of thought.

I have what is called a Methylation issue, which is one of the reasons that I got sick. This is an anomaly to my DNA and hinders my ability to detoxify. I need B-12 to Methylate – and the best way to get B-12 is from beef. I feel better when I eat meat – and now I understand why.

I am sensitive to soy, a major protein in Vegan diets, and I have Type II Diabetes, so eating a lot of beans for protein is not an option. (high in carbohydrates)

You will need to make your own decision. The key is, whether you eat meat or not, you should be consuming far more veggies in every color of the rainbow for optimal health. Make your plate 75% vegetable. (And that doesn't mean French fries)

Grass-Fed Beef

Let's start with beef, and what you need to know to eat clean.

I eat organic grass fed grass-finished beef unless I am in a situation where it is simply not available (most restaurants). So, what does this mean, and where do I shop?

To start, it means we don't go out much. And when we do, we tend to go to organic restaurants that make fun, gourmet vegetable dishes. In other words, I cook most of what I eat.

When I started on my journey, I was told to eat grass-fed beef, but I didn't know the grass-fed grass-finished part. If the cow is not grass-finished, he is fed grain at the end, to fatten him up and give him more marbleization for flavor. For anyone with gluten sensitivities, this is a problem. And if it is grass-fed and not organic and not grass-finished, likely the feed is GMO, so we are back to the toxic cocktail.

I try to eat organic meat. Grass-fed beef is defined by the USDA[250] as "organic livestock that must be:

- "Produced without genetic engineering, ionizing radiation, or sewage sludge.
- "Managed in a manner that conserves natural resources and biodiversity.
- "Raised per the National List of Allowed and Prohibited Substances (National List).
- "Overseen by a USDA National Organic Program – Authorized certifying agent, meeting all USDA organic regulations.
- "Fed 100 percent certified organic feed, except for trace minerals and vitamins used to meet the animal's nutritional requirements.
- "Managed without antibiotics, added growth hormones, mammalian or avian byproducts, or other prohibited feed ingredients (e.g., urea, manure, or arsenic compounds)."

Farmers and ranchers must accommodate the health and natural behavior of their animals year-round. For example, organic livestock must be:

- "Managed organically from the last third of gestation (mammals) or second day of life (poultry).
- "Allowed year-round access to the outdoors except under specific conditions (e.g., inclement weather).
- "Raised on certified organic land meeting all organic crop production standards.
- "Raised per animal health and welfare standards."
- I can buy organic grass-fed grass-finished organic beef at Whole Foods now several months of the year. You have to be careful because sometimes it states it is vegetarian finished and I don't eat that.

I can also buy 100% grass-fed beef at **Sprouts**, but it is from Ecuador or Bolivia, so I am not sure that their standards are the same. It certainly is better than eating factory farmed meat. Check around where grass-fed grass-finished beef is available in your neighborhood. There is an American Grass-fed Association[251], and you can search online for outlets for organic grass-fed grass-finished[252] beef in your area.

When I can't get my beef from **Whole Foods**, I buy from **Wellness Meats**[253] in MO online. The quality of their beef, pork, chicken, duck, etc. is excellent. They pay for shipping but add a $7.50 service charge per order. They do run a weekly sale, so I try and stock up on those items at point of sale.

Other advantages to eating grass-fed grass-finished organic beef.[254]

- In my opinion, grass-fed grass-finished beef tastes better. Some prefer the taste of the marbleized fat in conventional beef.
- The cow has eaten his natural diet his whole life, and all of that fiber passes to us when we eat grass-fed grass-finished beef.
- Grass-fed beef grass-finished has significantly higher Omega-3s, which is substantially better for us.
- Grass-fed beef grass-finished has more minerals and vitamins.
- Grass-fed beef is a great source of K-2.[255]
- Grass-fed beef grass-finished has more Beta-Carotine and CLA.
- Grass-fed beef grass-finished has less fat than factory farmed meat.
- Grass-fed Grass-finished beef is one of the best available sources of B-12.

Dr. Frank Lipman, MD wrote, in a blog on his **Be Well** website, an article called *Meat Smarts, 3 Ways To Get Healthy About Meat* (11/16/2016) – "... you always want to eat the happiest healthiest animal around."[256]

An article on the **Food Revolutions Network** website, called *"The Truth About Grass-Fed Beef"* states[257] "In addition to consuming less energy, (growing corn to feed factory farmed animals, consumes an enormous amount of energy) grass fed beef has another environmental advantage — it is far less polluting. The animals' wastes drop onto the land, becoming nutrients for the next cycle of crops. In feedlots and other forms of factory farming, however, the animals' wastes build up in enormous quantities, becoming a staggering source of water and air pollution."

The downside of Grass-fed beef grass-finished that amount of pasture land needed to grow the herd, and Grass-fed beef grass-finished creates a tremendous amount of methane gas, which is a factor in climate change.

Again, if you follow Dr. Hyman's advice, and eat Pagan, it is the best of all possible worlds.

Bison is an excellent alternative to beef. Buffalo are grass fed by nature, and the meat is delicious.

Chicken

I can't eat chicken, and I admit I miss it. After eating so much chicken in my life, free-range, pastured and just plain chicken, for some reason, I am now sensitive to it. I used to eat so much chicken that I joked I thought I was going to start to cluck at any moment. Now, out of the blue, it is a big sensitivity for me. Eliminating chicken from my diet has been a big step towards eliminating my pain.

And again, although I am not going to go into details, the way factory chickens are grown and treated is beyond gross. Their conditions are horrific. It's dreadful. The same goes for chicken eggs from chickens that are not pastured. Frightening. It makes me sick to my stomach.

And remember, all of those stress hormones pass directly from the bird into your body. You don't want them; so, eat organic chicken, only, ever.

So, let's talk about organic chickens and a few things that you can expect.

Whole Foods gives a number to their meats and chicken meat. You want a 4 or a 5.

Because these chickens get to live relatively naturally, then tend to be skinnier and cost a fortune because the farmer had to wait for the chicken to grow naturally. Buy this chicken anyway.

This is the explanation of the differences from the Whole Foods website.[258] "Step 4 is the first pasture-based Step. Birds at Step 4 live continuously on pasture or in foraging areas and are only housed at night or when seasonal conditions might put them at risk. Pasture is an area of grasses managed to provide nourishment as well as a mat of vegetation under their feet. A foraging area doesn't need to have grass but can include bushes and low trees that provide areas where the birds can nestle and not be visible to aerial predators. And, since chickens are descendants of Jungle fowl, this gives them the perfect environment to keep busy pecking, exploring and foraging for bugs!: Step 4 – Campo Lindo Farms, Pitman Family Farms, Shenandoah Valley Farms, and Vital Farms

"Steps 5 and 5+ are much more challenging to achieve. At Step 5, birds are bred to thrive in an outdoor environment and must be raised in small flocks. Several of our local suppliers have been able to reach this prestigious Step rating: Field to Family,

Petaluma Poultry, Pitman Family Farms and White Oak Pastures. For the highest Step level – Step 5+ – birds are bred, hatched and raised on the same farm. While there aren't yet Step 5+ chickens, some of our suppliers are already starting to explore this option. So, now you know a bit more about the ratings on the chicken in our fresh meat case."

Again, look at it as a condiment on your plate and you will be fine. You don't need more than that. The size of your palm or less.

If a chicken is truly pasture raised, with 10 meters of land for him to forage, he is much healthier, is high in omega-3s, is higher in total antioxidant nutrients, and all around better for you. He also tastes better.

20 years ago, I was traveling quite a bit to Thailand. I couldn't get over how delicious chicken was there. It was delicious because at that time, it was pasture raised. (Or most likely, backyard raised.)

All B vitamins are present in chicken meat, including B-1, B-2, B-3, B-5, B-6, B-12, folate, biotin, and choline.[259] A pastured chicken also has higher levels of alpha-linoleic acid and conjugated linoleic acid. A factory farmed chicken is fed synthetic vitamins because he cannot get them from his diet.

A pastured chicken includes insects in his diet which makes him taste better.

Mary's chicken is an excellent brand of pastured chicken. You can buy both level 4 and level 5 Mary's Chickens at Whole Foods. You can look up Mary's chicken online to find other stores that sell it.

Mary's also grows organic turkey. I do eat turkey, and often buy ½ a bird to make turkey soup, which is a favorite in my house. We also can get Diestel's free run pastured organic turkey, which is delicious. A ½ turkey is not inexpensive, but we get 2 meals just off the meat, and then about 10 meals off the soup, so it ends up being an economical choice.

Lamb

Sheep eat grass, so it is likely that lamb has been treated better all the way to your grocery store.

"Lambs live their whole lives on the farm, eating mostly hay and grass, using a sustainable grazing method that emulates their natural environment."[260]

Eating lamb also lowers your risk for cardiovascular disease.[261]

Ask your butcher if your lamb has been "finished" on grain. This could be a source for GMO's that you want to avoid.

Pork

You want organic pastured pork for the same reasons that you want organic pastured beef. The pig is treated humanely; he eats what he is meant to eat by nature, so he is healthier when he goes to butcher.

And you want the pork you buy to be organic for the same reasons as listed for organic beef. Otherwise, he grows in disgusting conditions, is fed synthetic vitamins, GMO feed, and given hormones and is an unhealthy choice.

If it's an option, heritage pork is a great choice. "Pork that comes from rarer breeds of pig that have been raised in humane and environmentally friendly conditions for a number of generations"[262] is called heritage pork.

Eggs

Only pastured chicken eggs. Period. The way little chicks are treated is disgusting, if not more disgusting, on factory farms as all of the poor factory farmed animals above.

I buy only Vital Farms eggs. They have several brands. They are even more humane treating the little male chicks that get born. I don't have access to pastured farm eggs directly from the farm, since I am a city girl. Vital Farms eggs are loaded with Omega-3's and healthier all the way around. Their "girls" get a change of scenery a couple of times a week and get to forage for their food, as God intended. If you have a farmers' market that you routinely visit, ask about how their chickens are treated and if they get to be outdoors (or protected at night if necessary) and whether they get to forage for their food.

Compared to other eggs these are expensive. However, my scrambled eggs in the morning, with fresh organic spinach, is about the same as an egg Mc Muffin (if I added in the English Muffin, which I don't eat because of gluten sensitivity) – and so, so much healthier.

Fish

In addition to the disgusting way that fish are farmed, there are other nasty chemicals used in the process. Fish factory farms are even threatening our natural fish supply interrupting what is found in nature.

"The overfishing of wild sardines, anchovies, mackerel, herring and other fish upsets natural ecosystems. We are not taking strain off wild fisheries," says agricultural economist Rosamond L. Naylor. "We are adding to it. This cannot be sustained forever."[263]

Again, farmed fish are fed growth hormones and grow as much as 6 times faster than wild fish. These hormones can screw up our wild fish and cannot be good in the long run. Farmed fish escape and breed with wild fish. The wild fish will not be able to overcome this disruption over time.

Wild fish is what you want to eat, especially wild salmon. (Atlantic salmon is farmed.) Wild salmon is an excellent source of Omega-3 fats. They are an excellent source of Vitamin D. Wild-caught salmon are healthy protein, and have selenium, niacin, vitamin B-12, phosphorus, magnesium and vitamin B6.[264]

The best fish to eat are:

- Wild-caught Alaskan salmon (canned or fresh) and wild caught sockeye salmon
- Mackerel
- Herring

Check EWG's list of best seafood to eat.[265] Their list includes:

- Sardines
- Rainbow trout
- Wild mussels (farmed are loaded with chemicals)
- Atlantic Mackerel
- Oysters
- Pollack

Shrimp

Most shrimp sold in our country is grown in factory farms in Thailand. The whole shrimp farming industry in Thailand is ugly. They use chemicals that are carcinogenic; they use child labor; they are polluting the waters which will long term, have ecological impact.

You should only buy shrimp that you know is wild.

We buy from our "fish" lady who has been in business for 30 years and her parents for 30 years before that. Her shrimp is wild from the Gulf of Mexico.

You can also ask for shrimp that is certified by an independent agency, such as the Wild American Shrimp or the Marine Stewardship Council. These certifications certify that wild fisheries are well-managed and sustainable.

If you cannot find these, then opt for wild-caught shrimp from North America. There are great shrimps available from the Gulf of Mexico and from the Pacific Northwest. I am not familiar with other parts of the country, but make sure you ask about what you are buying.

Alternatively look for the Best Aquaculture Practices label, which is for farmed (not wild) shrimp. This label means that the shrimp were raised without antibiotics and in conditions that exceed local environmental regulations.

Now, all of the choices I have given you above are more expensive. Eggs as the main course are not an expensive meal, even though you are paying a lot more for the dozen to ensure they are "happy" eggs. Smaller sizes of meat and fish are better for you. Remember, your body mostly needs nutrients from beautiful organic veggies. Make this a way of life, and your body will begin to heal itself, and you will be grateful that you are eating organic and healthy.

It feels good to feel good.

Chapter 15

Good and Bad Cooking Oils

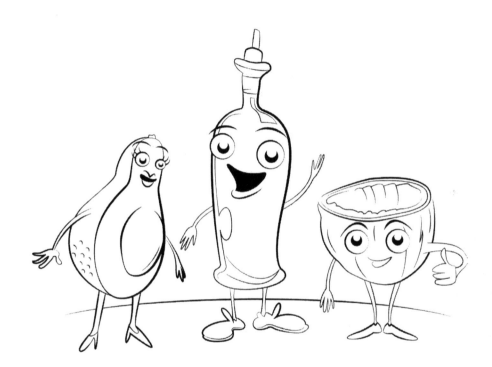

Dousing the flame of inflammation:

THE BIG TAKEAWAYS ON GOOD
AND BAD COOKING OILS

- Good oils were demonized by the vegetable oil industry and the sugar industry in major false news campaign starting in the 1960's. These campaigns have recently been proven false, and good oils are back in the limelight as a necessary food for health.
- DO NOT use vegetable oils, most are GMOs, and they are not good for you.
- Also, avoid Canola oil, it is all GMO and not good for you. This includes Canola-olive oil blends used in restaurants. Ask to see the bottle when you request it for your salad.
- The items on my Good Oil list are considered to be brain healthy, heart healthy, and necessary for healthy body function. They are also great for your skin, and they balance your hormones. Most of the Functional MDs that I follow strongly recommend you use these in your diet.
- Olive oil is a good choice for everything but cooking. It has a low smoke point which turns its good Omega-3's into Omega-6. Use Ghee, Coconut Oil or Grape Seed oil for cooking at higher heats, they are more stable and have a higher smoke point.
- Choose organic oil whenever possible.
- Smell your oils before using to ensure they have not gone rancid. Store them in a dark place.

Back in the 1970's, The Sugar Association, Coca-Cola, and candy manufacturers paid researchers at renowned universities (like Harvard) to produce studies that demonized the fat our grandparents ate, and to shed a positive light on sugar. There was no transparency and there were no facts to support the conclusions that these studies proclaimed. These studies became an example of false news that was widely reported and circulated. They changed the way America ate.

Marion Nestle, a professor of nutrition, food studies and public health at New York University, wrote an editorial accompanying the new paper in which she said the documents provided "compelling evidence" that the sugar industry had initiated research "expressly to exonerate sugar as a major risk factor for coronary heart disease."[267] These same studies demonized good fat to take the spotlight off of sugar.

In addition, there was another study published called **Dr. Key's Seven Countries Study** decades ago that examined heart risk based on lifestyle and dietary habits. Dr. Key's found "... that in the countries where people ate more fat — especially saturated fat — there were more cases of heart disease, and he concluded that the fat caused the disease." However, there is a difference between correlation and causation according to Dr. Mark Hyman, MD.[268]

The problem was when people ate less fat, they ate more carbohydrates and sugar. Since there was a study that falsely claimed sugar was good and fat was bad, our obesity epidemic was born.

What all of this did was to demonize what we now know are good fats:

- Butter
- Lard
- Tallow
- Coconut Oil
- Avocado oil
- Nut oils
- Flax seed oil
- Seeds oils
- Ghee
- Fatty wild fish.

There is a lot of current research released that shows that the good fats listed above, are not bad for us, but instead, they have many important uses in the body. These studies show that the fats above are good for us, and that they feed our body and our brain. These fats are actually necessary for healthy body function.[269]

For some reason, olive oil escaped being demonized, probably because it isn't saturated fat. But as a result of this demonization, a whole new generation of oils that were horrible for us were born in the 1960s.

Hydrogenated oils, Trans Fats, and Vegetable Oils, all of which are harmful to the body, filled the gap:

- Sunflower oil
- Safflower oil

- Corn oil
- Soybean oil
- Canola oil

These industries saw an opportunity and advertised how bad the saturated oils were, and how wonderful these vegetable oils were to replace them.

Between the false studies and the study that created an incorrect correlation, it was a perfect storm.

Many of these oils are now also genetically modified, making them an even greater health hazard. The new reality that these are harmful hasn't caught up yet with the public, restaurants, processed foods (which are loaded with tons of bad ingredients), salad dressings, etc., and it will be some time before they get discontinued because they are CHEAP.

Be very careful in restaurants by the way. What most restaurants call olive oil is a canola-olive oil blend. I state, that I am sensitive to canola oil, so I force the restaurant to show me the bottle. It is rarely real olive oil, but usually this connived blend oil. I try not to use or eat canola oil, ever. Canola oil is genetically modified and harmful to the body.

Canola oil was developed through conventional plant breeding from rapeseed. It was developed in Canada in the 1970s. In order to obtain drought resistant varieties genetically modified versions were introduced in 2011. I read a story that it got named because of its origin (Canada) and that it rhymed with Granola, making it sound healthy.

Canola oil has been shown to:[270]

- Cause liver and kidney problems.
- Cause heart disease because of the high Erucic acids in it.
- Has a correlation with Hypertension.
- Has a correlation with increased strokes.
- Increases heart disease because It is high in trans fats.

Canola also has all of the health side effects of other GMO crops.

I won't go deep into the trans-fat issue because it is pretty well known now, that they are unhealthy. Trans-fats are defined by Wikipedia as "vegetable fats for use in margarine, snack food, packaged baked goods and frying fast food starting in the 1950s. Trans-fat has been shown to consistently be associated, in an intake-dependent way, with increased risk of coronary heart disease, a leading cause of death in Western nations."[271]

As a child, butter vs. margarine was a continual debate. My Dad, a chemist, was annoyed that I wouldn't eat margarine. I hated the taste. My Mom had to buy butter just for me. We did monthly taste tests because my Dad swore I could not tell the difference … I always won. Who knew that my body instinctively knew what to eat. (Too bad it didn't stop me from eating excess sugar. Ha!)

So, let's get back to the good oils. There are many advantages of including these in your diet.

Good fats help the following functions in the body:

- They speed up your metabolism
- They are healthy for brain function
- They balance your hormones
- They help you have beautiful skin.
- They can help you lose weight

Low-fat items need to be eliminated from your diet. You can reread Chapter 12 on low-fat dairy, and get part of the gist of why. Beyond that, when Big Food eliminated good fats, they increased sugar and added processed ingredients, many of which are synthetic. These foods have little or no food value and fail to give your body nutrients that feed its body functions. The body starves on low-fat foods.

Dr. Susan Blum commented that to reduce inflammation, the oils that she recommends are Ghee, Coconut Oil, and Avocado oil. She stated "The only healthy fats that are specifically gut healing are ghee (contains the SCFA butyrate) and coconut oil (anti-candida), and for anti-inflammatory action, the omega's EPA/DHA/GLA, olive oil."[272]

If you are not fighting inflammation the list that I am seeing for fats from the Functional community is the following:

These are the Good Oils:

- Coconut Oil
- Avocado oil
- Nut oils
- Flax seed oil
- Seeds oils
- Ghee
- Fatty wild fish.
- Olive Oil
- Grapeseed oil
- MCT oil

We ate in a Paleo restaurant (brilliant food) in Sedona, AZ and they used brown rice oil. That was a new one. But it was yummy.

Just like the rest of your food, these need to come from organic sources. Preferably the butter needs to be made from raw dairy products from grass-fed grass-finished cows. Or buy organic. The lard and tallow need to come from pastured pigs and cows.

The nuts need to be organic too; otherwise, all of the chemicals in the growing process come right up the roots and into the nuts. It was hard to believe what I discovered the terrible things that are done to almonds. They are pasteurized by law in California (where most are grown), which means they either go through a steam process (good) or they are soaked in a chemical cocktail comprised of antifreeze and hydraulic fluid.[273] I found this hard to believe and totally gross. I will just note that in my opinion, you either need to buy them from a farmers' market where you know the farmer (and because of his size he is exempt from this law), or you need to buy them from nuts.com and get the ones from Spain where this regulation does not exist.

I have also listed an article in the endnotes that lists how your almonds have been treated by brand. Whole Foods, Trader Joes, and many others do not use the chemical bath. If you don't see what you are buying on the list, call corporate and ASK.

A couple of notes on the good fats

Olive Oil

The mafia has gotten involved in the olive oil industry and is cutting good olive oil with yukky vegetable oils. Buy Olive oil from one of the following sources:

- From a local farm at a farmers' market
- From California, where there is a law to protect that it is olive oil and nothing else
- From Italy where the Olive Industry organizations CIO and CIA certify with complete transparency what oils are in the bottle

Otherwise you don't know that the oil you bought as olive oil is actually olive oil.

California Olive Oil

In 2014 the California Olive Oil industry got a law passed to protect it.

"The California olive industry will now be able to distinguish itself as the authentic, premium-quality, extra virgin olive oil producer to American consumers," Jeff Columbini, chair of the OOCC said in a release. "Consumers will now be able to know that when they are purchasing and consuming California extra virgin olive oil, it truly is 100 percent extra virgin olive oil."[274]

The Italian Olive Oil followed, and created their CIA and CNO certification. They track the olive oil from the tree to the bottle to ensure it is only real Italian olive oil.

Things to know about the other "good" oils:

- Coconut Oil – Needs to be Virgin Unrefined. I buy from **Nutiva** when they have a special sale. Get on their mailing list.
- Avocado Oil[275] – I buy from **Thrive Market**, and I buy the Primal Kitchen brand I also use **Primal Kitchen Avocado Mayonnaise**. I also buy San Lucas avocado oil from California. I order it online.
- Speaking of Mayo, I also buy **Soy-free Vegenaise** by **Follow Your Heart**. This tastes just like Best Foods/Helmans to me. Love, it! I just saw that Thrive Market has a Coconut oil based Mayo. I look forward to trying it.

- Ghee, I buy from Thrive Market. There is a big saving over Whole Foods prices. I am sensitive to dairy, but since the milk fats are removed from Ghee, it doesn't bother me. I use it to cook with, bake with and to "butter" my toast. It's a lovely substitution for the butter which I can't have.
- **MCT oil** – Medium chain triglycerides. Look for MCT from Coconut. Great for your immune system, for your gut, for your brain. I use the one from **Bulletproof**. Bulletproof recommends you add just a bit to your hot morning beverage, especially coffee. There is a lot of buzz about this oil in the Paleo community.

Part 4
Toxins in Your Home and in Your Body

Chapter 16

Cosmetics

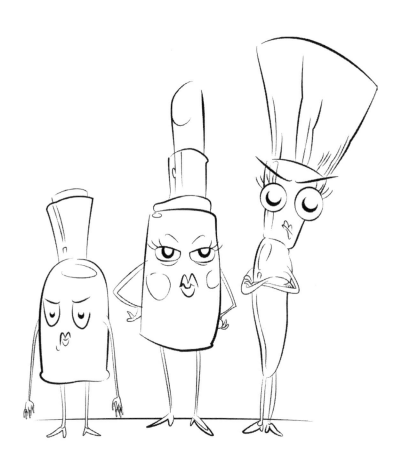

Dousing the flame of inflammation:

THE BIG TAKEAWAYS ON COSMETICS

- Beauty begins in the gut.
- Our skin is our largest organ, and our cosmetics are loaded with chemicals that are harmful to our body.
- Eliminating our toxic load is critical to healing our gut and quelling inflammation
- There is little regulation on cosmetic ingredients, so it is time to get educated.
- Look up what you are using on the Skin Deep database on EWG. If it's toxic, consider trying one of my recommendations, or search and find a cleaner brand to use.
- Stop using anything with fragrance. Change to essential oils in a clean carrier oil and make sure you buy from a source that is not selling synthetic oils. Use high quality essential oils as cologne, air fresheners, and any place where you used fragrances before.

Before we begin, the most important thing you can do for your body, your skin, your teeth, your nails and your hair is to heal your gut. Go back to my Chapter 4 on autoimmune disease to learn how to do that. Healing your gut will clear your acne, eliminate eczema, psoriasis, and it will help you have healthy hair, healthy nails, and a healthy attitude (which is part of beauty). There is no beauty product that can substitute for overall good health, and good health depends on a healthy biome. Remember, you are what you eat!

Go back and review to Part 3 on Food to understand more about how to do this. But each chapter in this book has to do with creating health, and doing that allows your beauty to shine through.

There are an incredible number of toxins lurking in your cosmetics and personal care products. Who knew? It doesn't matter if they are from the drug store (almost all toxic synthetic ingredients) or very expensive brands (still often loaded with toxins). Cosmetics are not regulated, and since our skin is our largest organ, what we are putting on our skin can be very detrimental to our health.

Cosmetics have never particularly been regulated.

Until recently, The Cosmetic Act of 1938 was the only guideline for the FDA. This law came about because mascara sold before 1938 had rat poison in it and blinded the consumer. According to Wikipedia, "Under the Act, the FDA does not approve cosmetic products, but because the Act prohibits the marketing of adulterated or misbranded cosmetics in interstate commerce, it can remove cosmetics from the market that contain unsafe ingredients or that are mislabeled. The FDA can and does inspect cosmetics manufacturing facilities to ensure that cosmetics are not adulterated." It counted heavily on the Cosmetic industry to monitor itself. Yikes!

That has been it for the last 80 years. Last year, a bill was finally passed to add some regulation to the cosmetic industry. ***The Personal Care Product Safety Act of 2015***. "Strong provisions in the bill would advance the FDA's ability to protect Americans' health by improving current law in the following areas:

- "Directing the FDA to assess the safety of a minimum of five cosmetics chemicals a year;
- "Requiring companies to register their facilities, products and ingredients with the FDA;
- "Requiring companies to comply with good manufacturing practices;
- "Closing labeling loopholes by requiring full ingredient disclosure for professional salon products and web-based sales of cosmetics; and
- "Giving the FDA mandatory recall authority to get unsafe products off the shelves."[277]

Bottom line, it is a start, but it doesn't do enough.

You have to take responsibility to do your own research for your own health, to keep the toxins out of your house and off of your skin. This government regulation is not going to protect you.

In an article from **Take Part Beauty and Its Beastly Secrets:** *The Toxic Truth About Cosmetics* by Linda Sharpe[278]

- "According to the Environmental Working Group, 89 percent of 82.000 ingredients used in personal care products have not been evaluated for safety by the FDA

- "In fact, the US federal government doesn't require any health studies or pre-market testing on personal care products
- "As a result, many cosmetics are thought to contain carcinogens, reproductive toxins, and other chemicals that may pose health risks
- "Up to 60% of what we put on our skin gets absorbed into the bloodstream

"It gets worse: the list of toxic additives present in many cosmetics is jaw-droppingly huge. U.S. researchers report that *one in eight* of the 82,000 ingredients used in personal care products are industrial chemicals. Harmful ingredients in your makeup drawer that should be avoided at all costs include (but are certainly not limited to): Butyl Acetate, Butylated hydroxytoluene, Coal tar, Cocamide DEA/lauramide DEA, Diazolidinyl Urea, Ethyl Acetate, Formaldehyde, Parabens (methyl, ethyl, propyl and butyl), Petrolatum, Phthalates, Propylene glycol, Siloxanes, Sodium Laureth/sodium laurel sulfate, Talc, Toluene, Triclosan, and Triethanolamine"[279]

Chemicals in sunscreens are particularly toxic and are threatening sea life and coral as well as the human body.[280]

"Thankfully, some organizations have made the process as pain-free as possible. **The Environmental Working Group** has a *Skin Deep* online database, where you can instantly check the safety of over 78,000 personal care products. The **Compact for Safe Cosmetics** has a useful FAQ titled '*What Should I Buy?*' And there's an iPhone app called '**Think Dirty'** that allows you to scan the barcode of a cosmetics or personal care product (in the store, before you buy it!), and rates it across three different categories: Carcinogenicity, Developmental & Reproductive Toxicity, and Allergies & Immunotoxicities."[281]

I have read varying comments that depending upon the products you are using; you could be exposed from anywhere of 15 of these toxins to 200. The toxic load to our bodies is overwhelming.

"Every day we use products that we think are safe, but the truth is that most of these products are NOT safe – and manufacturers don't have to tell us. Ever since 1938 – when the FDA granted self-regulation to the cosmetics industry – products can be marketed without government approval of ingredients, regardless of what tests show. Most of the chemicals used have not been tested for long-term toxic effects. In a typical day, you might be exposed to over 200 different chemicals, many of which are suspected of causing cancer or juggling hormones. EPA tests conclude that ingredients in shampoos, dyes, and other personal care products "may also be playing havoc with hormones that control reproduction and development."[282]

You must start reading the labels of the cosmetics and personal care products that you purchase. There is a list of "Terrible Touch-Me-Not" [283]Chemicals that have appeared in a variety of articles on the subject. These include:

"Alcohol, Isopropyl (SD-40): (rubbing alcohol) a very drying and irritating solvent and dehydrator that strips your skin's moisture and natural immune barrier, making you more venerable to bacteria, molds, and viruses. It is made from propylene, a petroleum derivative and is found in many skin and hair products, fragrance, antibacterial hand washes as well as shellac and antifreeze. It can act as a "carrier" accelerating the penetration of other harmful chemicals into your skin. It may promote brown spots and premature aging of the skin. A Consumer's Dictionary of Cosmetic Ingredients says it may cause headaches, flushing, dizziness, mental depression, nausea, vomiting, narcosis, anesthesia, and coma. Fatal ingested dose is one ounce or less.

"DEA (diethanolamine), MEA (Monoethanolamine) & TEA (triethanolamine): hormone-disrupting chemicals that can form cancer-causing nitrates and nitrosamines. These chemicals are already restricted in Europe due to known carcinogenic effects. In the United States, however, they are still used despite the fact that Americans may be exposed to them 10-20 times per day with products such as shampoos, shaving creams, and bubble baths. Dr. Samuel Epstein (Professor of Environmental Health at the University of Illinois) says that repeated skin applications ... of DEA-based detergents resulted in major increase in the incidence of liver and kidney cancer. The FDA's John Bailey says this is especially important since "the risk equation changes significantly for children."

"DMDM Hydantoin & Urea (Imidazolidinyl): just two of many preservatives that often release formaldehyde which may cause joint pain, skin reactions, allergies, depression, headaches, chest pains, ear infections, chronic fatigue, dizziness, and loss of sleep. Exposure may also irritate the respiratory system, trigger heart palpitations or asthma, and aggravate coughs and colds. Other possible side effects include weakening the immune system and cancer.

"FD&C Color Pigments: synthetic colors made from coal tar, containing heavy metal salts that deposit toxins into the skin, causing skin sensitivity and irritation. Absorption of certain colors can cause depletion of oxygen in the body and death. Animal studies have shown almost all of them to be carcinogenic.

"Synthetic Fragrances: mostly synthetic ingredients can indicate the presence of up to four thousand separate ingredients, many toxic or carcinogenic. Symptoms reported to the FDA include headaches, dizziness, allergic rashes, skin discoloration, violent coughing and vomiting, and skin irritation. Clinical observation proves fragrances can affect the central nervous system, causing depression, hyperactivity, irritability, inability to cope, and other behavioral changes.

"Alternative – Organic Essential Oils.

"Mineral Oil: petroleum by-product that coats the skin like plastic, clogging the pores. Interferes with skin's ability to eliminate toxins, promoting acne and other disorders. Slows down skin function and cell development, resulting in premature aging. Used in many products such as baby oil, which is 100% mineral oil!

"Alternatives – Moisture Magnets (Saccharide Isomerate) from beets; Ceramides, Jojoba, and other vegetable oils, etc.

"Polyethylene Glycol (PEG): potentially carcinogenic petroleum ingredient that can alter and reduce the skin's natural moisture factor. This could increase the appearance of aging and leave you more vulnerable to bacteria. Used in cleansers to dissolve oil and grease. It adjusts the melting point and thickens products. Also, used in caustic spray-on oven cleaners.

"Propylene Glycol (PG) and Butylene Glycol: gaseous hydrocarbons which in a liquid state act as 'surfactant' (wetting olagents and solvents). They easily penetrate the skin and can weaken protein and cellular structure. Commonly used to make extracts from herbs. PG is strong enough to remove barnacles from boats! The EPA considers PG so toxic that it requires workers to wear protective gloves, clothing, and goggles and to dispose of any PG solutions by burying them in the ground. Because PG penetrates the skin so quickly, the EPA warns against skin contact to prevent consequences such as brain, liver, and kidney abnormalities. But there isn't even a warning label on products such as stick deodorants, where the concentration is greater than in most industrial applications.

"Alternatives – water extracted herbs, Therapeutic Essential Oils, etc.

"Sodium Lauryl Sulfate (SLS) & Sodium Laureth Sulfate (SLES): detergents and surfactants that pose serious health threats. Used in car washes, garage floor cleaners, and engine degreasers – and in 90% of personal-care products that foam. Animals exposed to SLS experience eye damage, depression, labored breathing, diarrhea, severe skin irritation, and even death. Young eyes may not develop properly if exposed to SLS because proteins are dissolved. SLS may also damage the skin's immune system by causing layers to separate and inflame. When combined with other chemicals, SLS can be transformed into nitrosamines, a potent class of carcinogens. Your body may retain the SLS for up to five days, during which tie it may enter and maintain residual levels in the heart, liver, the lungs, and the brain.

"Alternative – Ammonium Cocoyl Isethionate.

"Triclosan: a synthetic 'antibacterial' ingredient – with a chemical structure similar to Agent Orange! The EPA registers it as a pesticide, giving it high scores as a risk to both human health and the environment. It is classified as a chlorophenol, a class of chemicals suspected of causing cancer in humans. Its manufacturing process may produce dioxin, a powerful hormone-disrupting chemical with toxic effects measured in the parts per trillion; that is only one drop in 300 Olympic-size swimming pools! Hormone disruptors pose enormous long-term chronic health risks by interfering with the way hormones perform, such as changing genetic material, decreasing fertility and sexual function, and fostering birth defects. It can temporarily deactivate sensory nerve endings, so contact with it often causes little or no pain. Internally, it can lead to cold sweats, circulatory collapse, and convulsions. Stored in body fat, it can accumulate to toxic levels, damaging the liver, kidneys, and lungs and can cause paralysis, suppression of immune function, brain hemorrhages, and heart problems. Tufts University School of Medicine says that triclosan is capable of forcing the emergence of 'super bugs' that it cannot kill. Its widespread use in popular antibacterial cleaners, toothpaste, and household products may have nightmare implications for our future."

Other Common Toxic Ingredients To Avoid:

- Aluminum
- Phthalates
- DEET
- Dioxins
- Formaldehyde
- PABA
- Para-Aminobenzoic Acid (PABA)
- Parabens
- Phenoxyethanol
- Toluene
- Camphor

EWG has a new database called *SKIN DEEP*. You can literally look up the products that you are using, and see their rating, with one being the safest, and ten being the most toxic. If your product is not in the database, which includes 64,400+ products, you can look up the ingredients.

This is evolving. I chose new cosmetics four years ago, and after buying multiple products to see what worked for me, I am discovering that a few of my picks now also have some toxic ingredients. As I am writing this chapter, I am looking up ingredients again; I am re-evaluating some of the items I am using. I will put a list of the brands I use by category in this chapter, to give you a place to start, but these are items that work for me. Each of us is unique, so you may want to make other choices. I will also provide links to make your research easier.

EWG recently started a certified program called *EWG Verified.*[284]

What does EWG VERIFIED™ mean?

Among other things, products must:

- Be free of **EWG's** ingredients of concern
- Fully disclose all ingredients

My suggested products would be another place to start. There are also recommendations on the **Safe Cosmetics.org** site.

It is imperative that you take control of what you are putting on your body. I am asking you to spend time and to do the research because it's incredibly important to your health.

It's even more important, if you have a teenage daughter, to know what chemicals she is using on her body.[285] Many of these toxic chemicals dangerously disrupt hormones, causing premature puberty and can trigger lasting long-term health issues, weight issues, and disease.[286]

I recommend you look up each product you are currently using and that you take a second look in a couple of years.

I am about to recommend many products that I have found work well for me. This is just a place to get you started. You are unique, so these may not be perfect for you. If that is the case, you will need to start your own research. Understand that I am not making any money on these suggestions. I offer these recommendations to you as to help you start your own journey to wellness.

THINGS I LEARNED BY PRODUCT CATEGORY

POWDERS

Powders can cause an inhalation risk. The product that I use over my base, and also as my blush, does not cause that issue.

I recommend **W3ll People**, whose products are a "1" on the **EWG** scale, and *verified EWG Safe*.

MAKEUP BASE

This is an area where I am about to make a change.

Although the original product that I chose is a "5" on the EWG scale and gives my older skin good coverage, I have discovered that it has a chemical in it that is a "9", Retinyl Palmitate, and then the rest of the ingredients are a "3" or less. Not acceptable. I use the **W3ll People Narcissist Foundation Stick** as a concealer (*EWG verified*, and when I looked it up, it is a "1"), I am now going back to the drawing board to find a base that isn't poisoning my body.

I am just trying a liquid base from **Vapour ...** I am adding a little concealer that comes from W3ll people, and now I get good coverage for my older skin.

On the cosmetic site for the product that I now find unacceptable, it states. Free of parabens, mineral oil, petrolatum, and phthalates,

Which I am sure is all true. The stamps above seem impressive. However, you must be vigilant and look up all of your products, no matter what the company tells you. The Retinyl Palmitate used in this product is a deal breaker for me.

I wrote to this company and questioned the Retinyl Palmitate. They haven't responded. This product is sold at Whole Foods and Sprouts. Don't be fooled. Look your choices up.

From the EWG database:

"Health Concerns of the Ingredient (Retinyl Palmitate)**:**

"Overall Hazard is high (the bad ingredient that is a '9')

"Developmental & reproductive toxicity is also high

"Other **HIGH concerns:** Biochemical or cellular level changes; Other **LOW concerns:** Data gaps, Ecotoxicology, Organ system toxicity (non-reproductive)

"About RETINYL PALMITATE (VITAMIN A PALMITATE): Retinyl palmitate is an ingredient composed of palmitic acid and retinol (Vitamin A). Data from an FDA study indicate that retinyl palmitate when applied to the skin in the presence of sunlight, may speed the development of skin tumors and lesions. FDA, Norwegian, and German health agencies have raised a concern that daily skin application of vitamin A creams may contribute to excessive vitamin A intake for pregnant women and other populations.

"Function(s): Skin-Conditioning Agent – Miscellaneous; SKIN CONDITIONING

"Synonym(s): RETINYL PALMITATE, AXEROPHTHOL PALMITATE; HEXADECANOATE RETINOL; RETINOL PALMITATE; RETINOL, HEXADECANOATE; VITAMIN A PALMITATE; AQUASOL A; AROVIT; OPTOVIT-A; RETINOL PALMITATE; VITAMIN A PALMITATE"

Enough said!!!!

MASCARA

This was one of the first categories where I had a sensitivity reaction. After trying dozens of mascaras, including mascaras that were touted as Hypoallergenic, I settled on **Blinc**, which coats the eyelash with little tubes. I still use **Blinc**; my body is not sensitive to it. It is a four on the **EWG** research, and there is something in it that is a "6". I recommend the **W3ll People** mascara that is a "1" and is *EWG verified*. If something is bothering you, listen to your body. Let it vote. There are alternatives.

BLUSH

I use **W3ll People** a "1" on the **EWG** scale. It gives me great color, but not too much. I love the colors it comes in. It is affordable. Their products are now available at Target online as well as online at their own website.

W3ll People offers small samples on their website for a minimal price so that you can try their cosmetics before you take a full-size leap. Kudos to the company for that!!!

(My new find **Vapour** also offers small samples, which is terrific.)

SKIN CARE

This category took me a lot of time and trial and error before I settled on a line that I love. **Keys-Soap**, this company was born when the wife got skin cancer and suddenly all products irritated her skin. Her husband was a biochemist in Silicon Valley, and he quit his job to develop a line that she could use. Their products are amazing, and they are all a "1" on the EWG scale. I use their skin cream, their eye cream, and then expanded to their shampoo, their facial wash, and their body wash.

My scalp had been itchy for more than 25 years. Who'd of thunk that I was sensitive to the ingredients in my shampoo? Now that I done the research, I know that shampoos are loaded with chemicals. **Key's** products are clean.

Key's products are also way more affordable than the expensive toxic "beauty" creams that I used on my skin for years. If you buy from their website, you can also bundle products for a discount.

You can also buy them on **Amazon**.

They also have expanded to a product line for Dogs which I understand are amazing. (Although, I love all animals, I own cats. *smile*)

Most recently they have introduced products to take the place of anything in your medicine cabinet that has petroleum in it. They are fantastic. I discuss this further in my Chapter 18 on over the counter drugs and products.

The best thing about **Key's** is you can also order samples on their website for a nominal fee and see if they work for you. More kudos for them!!!

DEODORANT

This has been another perplexing category for me. I started having an extreme reaction to deodor*ants* over 25 years ago. Some gave me a rash; others made me raw.

There are many products now to choose from, but five years ago, after years of struggle, I read an article in **Bazaar Magazine** about a new line of products by a woman with Lupus who started developing an underarm deodorant out of self-defense. I love it and have used it ever since. It is now on the *Clean Cosmetic* recommended product list.

Soapwalla[287], the deodorant cream is $14 and lasts a very long time. There is also a $5 sample size available on their website Yeah! It comes in two fragrances (essential oils). And best of all, it works! It is now available at Target, Walmart, and Amazon. It is listed on **SafeCosmetics.org** as a win.

FRAGRANCES

I hate to tell you this, but they are very toxic. What makes it worse is you are using fragrance on your skin, and all of these toxins get absorbed. Most of the ingredients are synthetic, and there are 4000 of them that are harming your body. Some go so deep that your body can't detox them out of the body, so they stick around for the long haul.

"Most 'fragrances' are synthetic, petroleum-based and toxic to our bodies, capable of triggering skin problems, allergies, respiratory difficulties, hormonal, metabolic and thyroid problems, even certain cancers and neurological damage."[288]

There are currently studies being done to see if these toxic chemicals are a cause of Alzheimer's and Parkinson's disease. Until the studies are in, my recommendation is that you stop using them and throw them away.

I actually have a funny story about fragrance. A few years ago, when I started dating again, I went out with a guy that had doused himself in cologne. Before we even got to dinner, I asked that he take me home. I couldn't breathe. We scheduled another date. But when he returned, he still was doused in cologne, even though he knew my sensitivity. When I asked why, he told me that he had never had a woman tell him he took her breath away. Needless to say, the date was over, and I never saw him again.

Shortly after that, I started to have a big problem with fragrance in fabric softeners. I would wake up in the morning with my lips all swollen and again, it was hard to breathe. So, I eliminated fragrances long before I had the symptoms of autoimmune disease.

This is why I was reacting:

In an article by Dr. Frank Lipman MD called *"Fragrance Stinks"* March 2009[289]

"Fragrances Are Mysterious Chemical Cocktails

"Identifying individual chemicals that make up a particular fragrance is, unfortunately, virtually impossible for consumers. Why? Because manufacturers aren't required to list every ingredient in their proprietary fragrance brews. Instead of being called out on the label, questionable ingredients get to hide behind the word 'fragrance.' So, as far as the maker is concerned, it's all good. Like the catch-all phrase, 'natural flavors' that often appears on processed food labels, 'fragrance' is used to similar effect, keeping corporate secrets safe and consumers at risk. And that just stinks.

"Think of Fragrance as a Toxic Layer Cake

"According to consumer advocates the Environmental Working Group, over the course of the average day, women are exposed to more than 160 chemicals *just from their cosmetics alone*. Add to that, a few shower products, hair products, cleaning products and a load of laundry or two, and the amount of daily chemical exposure climbs even higher. The EWG also reported that tests of fragrance ingredients have found an average of 14 hidden compounds per formulation, including ones linked to hormone disruption and sperm damage. Multiply every scented product you use daily by a factor of 14, all that voluntary exposure to toxins starts to look like sheer madness."

This means you need to consider eliminating all products that have fragrance in them. Your perfumes and colognes are just the tip of the iceberg. Consider your detergents, your fabric softeners, the fragrances in your cosmetics, air fresheners, everything. They are all doing you harm.

So, what to use instead:

- I have a diffuser and use nonsynthetic essential oils to make my home smell fresh.
- I use a little of my favorite essential oils in a carrier oil and use it instead of perfume.

Beware of "fragrance oils." They are most likely harmful synthetics.

LIPSTICK

This category was frightening for me, because for 40 years, I have been known for my red lips. Guess what? Red lipstick is usually loaded with lead. (I am in the process of chelating toxic metals from my body, and yep, I am loaded with lead.)

So, what to do? The brand I was using was touted as one of the best lipsticks available on the market. It was loaded with hazardous ingredients.

So, after trying dozens of products, I landed on three that I thought were ok. Today I am knocking one off of my list due to one highly toxic ingredient.

I recommend

Elixery and **Lavera**. Both make very nice reds that stay in place and don't dry out my lips.

If these don't work for you, check back to the EWG Skin Deep Website.

NAIL POLISH

First of all, I have had acrylic nails for 40 years. I was a nail biter, and in spite of all of the psychological articles written about why someone bites their nails, I can tell you I was a nail biter because my nails were very weak, and when they got rough they annoyed me, so I chewed on them to smooth them out. Hark, acrylic nails were my solution. But acrylic nails are also extremely toxic, both during the process of having them put on and then on my body.

I found two nail polish companies that had less toxic products, so I have been using them (but I realize I am fooling myself), since I didn't want to give up the acrylics (toxic fumes and toxic chemicals.)

In the meantime, in my search for health, in the last year, I am using a lot of bone broth in my cooking, I realized when I took my fake nails off, my nails underneath were much harder, so I now am in the process of growing out my own nails. Yippee!

I have also started using **BioSil** for my hair and nails. Between the bone broth and the silica, I have hard nails for the first time in my life. Wowzie!

For nail polish, I chose the following brands. **Zoya** and **Sugar Loom**. Most nail polishes carry a toxic chemical called TPHP[290], which is an endocrine disrupter. Particularly dangerous to teenage girls, but also toxic for adults

SUNSCREEN

Another nasty category, loaded with toxins.

- Pick products with Zinc Oxide or Titanium dioxide as the active ingredient.
- Avobenzone at 3%
- Choose 30 SPH for intense sum
- Apply liberally and often
- Stay in the shade; wear hats in the mid-day sun. [291]

Truth In Aging wrote an article about the findings by **EWG** for the best sunscreens *called EWG's picks for best sunscreens and moisturizers with SPF*. They state:

"**EWG** tested 902 sunscreens and SPF moisturizers by running ingredient lists from manufacturers through extensive databases to evaluate their active components. Of these, only 5% met the EWG's criteria (which includes broad-spectrum protection from both UVA and UVB rays, stability of the formula, and safety of the individual ingredients)."[292]

They list all of **EWG**'s best findings by category, so I suggest you go to the article and use it as a guide.

Food Babe also did an article on her recommendations. *The Ingredients in Sunscreen Destroying Your Health*[293] See the endnote for her recommendations.

My choice is on the recommended list by EWG. Keys-soaps **Solar Rx Cosmetic Moisturizing Sunblock SPF 30**.

If you want to read all of EWG's concerns about sunscreens, read their article *Eight Little-Known Facts About Sunscreens* on their website. Remember, sunscreens go on your skin, so it is especially important to protect yourself from chemicals.

TOOTHPASTE

I have only recently solved this. Mint is a food sensitivity for me, so I can't use mint toothpaste. What is important is to avoid Triclosan, an endocrine disruptor, and carrageenan, which has been tested as a carcinogen.

My picks are:

- **DR. Brite** fluoride free Mineral toothpaste which is *EWG Verified*
- And **Miessence** Lemon Toothpaste which is a one on the **EWG** scale. (I use the lemon, but I am not crazy about the taste. Try the Mint)

When you do your research, you may find others that use mint. I also avoid Xylitol, a sugar alcohol that acts like a laxative on my body, but it doesn't seem to affect everyone that way. The **DR. Brite** does have it as an ingredient, but my body is saying it is ok in the small amounts I use in their toothpaste. Let your body vote on whether it can handle that ingredient or not.

Two other products that have helped me immensely:

BIOSIL

It is a silica product that I started using when lost a little hair one day washing my hair. I know that as we age, we do lose some hair, but not if I can help it. My hairdresser recently told me that my hair is not as thick as it used to be. When I gasped, he pointed out that I still have more hair than his other clients. But since my mother's hair got thin as she aged, I don't want to go there. Well, I believe BioSil will help me along the way. I think it's also partially responsible for my harder nails. My husband started using it, after he had lost some hair, and now he has a little fuzz starting to grow on his forehead. His hair cutter just commented that he is growing new hair. Win!

Catalase[294]

This is a new supplement from my favorite functional pharmacist, Suzy Cohen. Buy it from her website. It's great for hair and skin and helps the liver.

IN CONCLUSION

I have listed many resources and articles below that you can use to start your own investigation. I highly recommend that you start to clean up the toxic products you are using on and in your body. Again, this is a process. Decide upon new products one at a time. At least, when it is time to replace a product, pick something nontoxic at that point. Interestingly enough, many of these products are not as expensive as what I was previously using. Each step you take is a step closer to better health.

Chapter 17

Drinking Water

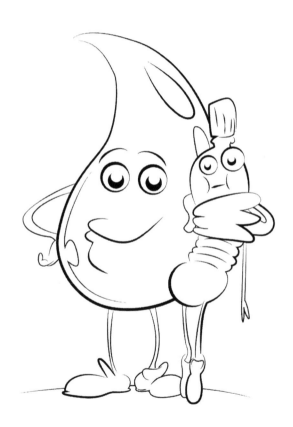

Dousing the flame of inflammation:

THE BIG TAKEAWAYS ON DRINKING WATER

- Water is essential to all body functions. How much water is the right amount of water?
- Be vigilant and find out what's in your water.
- Most of our tap water is loaded with contaminants,
- You need to buy a filter to remove the toxins.
- Bottled water is generally worse that your tap water.

How much water does your body need to thrive?

In a report issued by Ocean Robbins, an activist for nutrition, environmentalism, and animal rights, called *The Truth About Drinking Water and What You Need to Know to be Safe,* 11/22/2016 he states:

"Water is essential for life. Our bodies are 60% water, and without water, our bodies will die in just a few days. Every single cell, tissue, and organ in your body needs water to function."[296]

Every day, water:[297]

- Delivers oxygen to your body
- Nourishes your body's cells
- Nourishes your skin
- Flushes out toxins
- Aids in a healthy digestion
- Lubricates the eyes
- Is important for blood, and for muscles
- Lubricates the joints
- Allows chemical reactions in the body
- Breaks down your food for nutrition
- Protects your vital organs.
- Water is thought to help prevent cancer.
- Water hydrates your body.
- Water reduces fatigue.
- Water improves mood.

- Water improves digestion.
- Water flushes out toxins.

Water has no calories; drinking a lot of water through the day does the body lots of good. You need to drink the right amount. I have read that it is important to drink your body weight divided by two in ounces a day. That ended up being rather excessive for me, so I now try to drink about 70 ounces of water throughout the day. Drinking too much water can dilute essential electrolytes in your body. Listen to your body.

To make water alkaline, I squeeze a little lemon into my water. I love the taste, and lemon adds vitamin C, potassium, folate, B-6, Thiamin, and magnesium to my water, all good.

According to Dr. Josh Axe DNM, DC, CNS[298], in his paper on the **Benefits of Lemon Water: Detox Your Body and Skin**, adding a little lemon to your water:

- "Aids in digestion and detoxification
- "Bumps up the Vitamin C Quotient
- "Rejuvenates your skin and heals your body
- "Helps shed pounds
- "Boosts your energy and mood."

So, what's the problem drinking water from your tap? Your water could be poisoning you. The Flint, Michigan issue is not unique to them, although it is exasperated there.

Bottled Water does not solve the issue and might actually make it worse. So, let's take a look first at tap water and then look at bottled water and discuss the contaminants in each and what to do about them.

DEFINING THE TOXICITY PROBLEM

What comes out of your faucet?

The water you are drinking could be loaded with toxic chemicals. More research has been done since I first studied this for myself, and although the filter that I have on my drinking water helps, it does not screen out all of the toxins that could be present.

For starters, if it comes from a municipal source, the water that comes out of your tap is tested. The report is published in a place where you should be able to find it and take a look. I had to call my city to find it, but it should be available somewhere online.

You can also go to **EWG** (the Environmental Working Group) and check their database on your cities water. **EWG's _National Tap Water Atlas_** is found at www. ewg.org/tap-water

Remember Erin Brockovich? She was the activist made famous by Julia Roberts in the movie of the same name. The movie was about a how she went after industry (PG & E) to clean up the drinking water of a small California town because everyone in the town was getting horribly ill. Well, that chemical was Chromium-6, and it is present in 75% of America's water. Isn't that a ducky thought?

Beyond that, when **EWG** (the Environmental Working Group, which I encourage you to become very familiar with and I encourage you to support their research) tested tap water all around the country and discovered as many as 312 contamin*ants* and as many as 202 of these contamin*ants* are not regulated. President Bush's EPA Administration listed these contamin*ants* in our drinking water as one of the top 4 public health risks.[299] They include:

- Fluoride
- Arsenic
- Lead which can cause learning disabilities in children and hypertension in adult males
- Trihalomethanes which may cause bladder and rectal cancer
- Chromium-6 (Erin Brockovich target)
- Perchlorate
- Asbestos
- Mercury
- VOCS
- Industrial solvents
- Fuel Propell*ants*

- Antimony which is a byproduct of the petroleum in our ground
- Atrazine which is an herbicide sprayed on our crops that are sprayed with Glyphosate for a double toxic cocktail that is getting into our ground water and causing damage to the human reproductive system. This is found in 90% of the tap water tested.
- Additional Endocrine disrupters – residues of Pharmaceuticals', birth control medications, and hormones. Some scientists think that these Endocrine disruptors pose a greater threat to mankind than climate change.
- There are also residues of fertilizers found in our drinking water.

If you have a well, please get it tested.

In a report from the EPA on Dec 15, 2016[300], *In Reversal, EPA Confirms That Fracking Pollutes Drinking Water* the conclusion of the scientists studying the toxic effects of fracking stated "The report found that drinking water can be contaminated by spills of chemical-laced fracking fluid or wastewater, improper disposal of wastewater, and leakage from faulty well casings. It also said water supplies were threatened by the use of huge volumes of water to frack in drought-stricken areas." These chemicals have entered the water supplies in Pennsylvania, Wyoming, Texas, and Colorado, as well as other states that have permitted fracking.

Ok then. Should we be drinking bottled water that comes in plastic? What is in plastic bottles of water?

We spend a fortune on water in plastic bottles. The water in plastic bottles is estimated to cost 1900 times more than tap water. However, it is estimated that up to 44% of bottled water is tap water, just bottled in plastic. (Who knew? I certainly didn't.)

In an article in **Natural News** *Bottled Water Found Contaminated with Medications, Fertilizer, Disinfection Chemicals* 4/4/2009 they state: "EWG notes that while municipal water companies are required to test tap water yearly and disclose the results, there is no comparable requirement for the bottled water industry. Bottled water companies do not have to test their water or reveal the results when they do; they are not even required to tell consumers where the water came from or how it has been treated. A separate EWG survey of 228 bottled water brands found that less than half revealed their water's source or treatment history in their promotional materials."[301]

Dr. Josh Axe states in an article on his website called ***Tap Water Toxicity***

"Sam's Choice and **Gi**ants **Acadia** had a known carcinogen high enough to violate California law.[302]

"One of the leading brands increased breast cancer by 78%."[303]

"In a study of 10 leading brands of bottled water; **EWG** found 38 toxic pollut*ants* overall with each brand containing an average of 8 toxins.

"The chemicals they found included arsenic, chlorine byproducts, fertilizer, fluoride, fuel propell*ants*, heavy metals, industrial solvents, pharmaceutical drugs, plasticizers and radioactive isotopes. Four of these leading brands also contained bacteria."[304]

In a different article called ***Estrogen Epidemic: What's in Your Water?*** Dr. Axe states:

"25% of the bottled water purchased is tap water from **Coca-Cola** and **PepsiCo**.[305]

"Up to 44% of bottled water is just tap water. It may or may not be filtered. Bottled water is not regulated, and they are not required to publish their water quality tests."[306]

But the plastic bottles are toxic on their own, made with Bisphenol A, and Phthalates, which are endocrine disrupters that possibly increase breast, prostate, and ovarian cancers. In animal studies, they decrease sperm count and alter menstrual cycles.[307] Adult liver toxicity, heart disease, and diabetes may all be linked to BPA.

All of this is even more damaging to small children, whose cells are still undergoing genetic programming.[308]

When the plastic bottles get heated (like in a hot car, or in a microwave) they leach even more chemicals into the water.

For a moment in time, we were told that some numbers embossed on our plastic bottles were safe. Now they know that those bottles just have different unsafe chemicals in them.[309]

And I haven't even addressed all of the harm that all this plastic is doing to our planet.

These are all very frightening statistics. So, what do we do about it?

Solutions to get rid of the toxins

These are all beginning steps, but I believe that they will make a difference in your health.

I also want to encourage you to be your own advocate. Dig deeper into the subject. Get a copy of what is in your water. Get recommendations from the person running your water department. Call companies selling filters and pick their brains for what their product does.

I am lucky. I live in a city in Southern California that has its own water supply from the mountains that are to our north. We have natural artisan wells below our city. So, our water is relatively clean. None the less, I have a filter on my kitchen sink, and that is the water that I drink at home.

My long-term dream is to put a carbon filter water system on my entire home. Since skin is our largest organ, the chemicals that are in our water are being absorbed every day in the shower and the bathtub. The contaminants are also in the steam as you wash your dishes. But take one step at a time. Every step you take to rid your home of toxins is a step in the right direction.

Tap Water

Water Filter types and what I use.

Carbon filters, come both as a pitcher, and also tap-mounted. These are affordable and do remove common contaminants, like lead, and the by-products of the disinfection process. I use **Aquasana,** and mine is tap-mounted.

Aquasana's website states NSF Certified Claryum filtration technology independently tested and proven to remove over 97% of chlorine and chloramines. Also, reduces:

- Heavy metals like lead and mercury
- Chlorine resistant cysts like giardia and cryptosporidium
- Organic chemicals like herbicides, pesticides, and VOCs
- Pharmaceuticals like estrone and ibuprofen

They post a long list of different contaminants that are reduced up to 95%

If you can afford it, install a reverse osmosis system. These systems remove contaminants like arsenic and perchlorate. **Aquasana** declares that their system is 5 times more effective at removing toxins and contaminants. They have applied for certification from the NFS that this system also removes Chromium 6.

Both types of water systems have filters that need to be replaced. I am on an automatic system where my filters come by mail, and we change them.

If you choose reverse osmosis, then research any known health issues. They are such efficient systems that they strip the good minerals as well as the bad out of your water.

I recently received an email from Ocean Robbins (of the Baskin Robbins family turned environmental and food activist), that he had discovered a new system for removing toxins from water – a new Reverse Osmosis system, called the **AquaTru**. They might be worth looking into as a way to remove toxins from your water at home.

There are other expensive, complex water systems that not only remove contaminants but also turn the water alkaline and then reserve the acid water residue for cleaning. You would need to do your own research in this area. Although I drink my 70 ounces of water daily with lemon, to help it be slightly alkaline, some experts like Dr. Andrew Weil suggest that it is unnecessary, the human body is smart, and converts its own liquids to its perfect ph.[310] Other experts are vehement that alkaline is critical to a healthy body and to deterring cancer. Do your own research and then decide. (I have a close friend that swears by their waters system that separates the alkaline water from the acidic water. Along with an alkaline diet, she swears by the health benefits that she and her husband have had. You decide.)

Remember to drink filtered water, and also to cook with filtered water.

EWG lists many filtering systems. Do your own research, and choose what works with the contaminants in your water and what fits your budget.

Bottled Water

Ok, this is even more complex. We have become dependent on plastic bottles of water, and we take them with us everywhere. Now understanding that the water is often tap water, that it is not regulated, and that the plastic leaches chemicals into the water, what do we do?

I started buying the brand "**Real Water**" in glass bottles. I refill these bottles every day with my filtered water out of my tap. I take them into my office. I drink from them while I watch TV. Although these bottles are more expensive initially, they have saved me tons of money. I reuse the bottles, and they eliminate some plastic toxins and the water filter eliminates toxins in the tap water used in the bottles.

(These glass bottles are currently not in stock at Whole Foods. I called Real Water. The glass bottles are not available all year. Right now (Jan 17) they are in production. They are expected to hit the shelves in March. Real Water seems to think that their plastic bottle are safe, but they are made of PET plastic, which has recently been discovered to not be safe. Be forewarned.)

You can also buy cylinder glass bottles from Aquasana. I like their cylinder bottles with the blue caps. These work well in my car as they fit into the cup holder.

But the problem with glass bottles is fear of breakage. I just bought two stainless steel bottles from **Aquasana** to avoid the glass. They were not inexpensive, but will replace expensive plastic bottle of water for years. Win!

Make sure that you wash your bottles daily. I have a bottle brush that I wash them with, and then pop them into my dishwasher.

So, what do you do if you are traveling, and don't have access to your filtered water? Dr. Axe suggests buying spring water and filling up your glass bottles using that. He also suggests that you never buy plastic bottled water from a soft drink company.

Chapter 18

Drugs

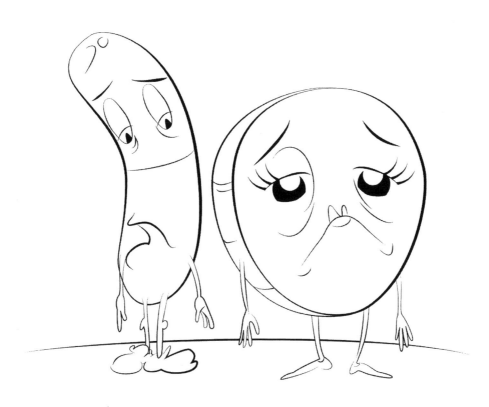

Dousing the flame of inflammation:

THE BIG TAKEAWAYS ON DRUGS

- Replace the over the counter drugs in your medicine cabinet with my suggestions below. Over the counter drugs have serious side effects.
- Stop using Petroleum Jelly products and replace them with the items suggested below.
- Build a new medicine cabinet with my suggestions below, with items your body can thrive on.
- Buy a copy of Drug Muggers Rodale Books; (February 15, 2011).by Suzy Cohen, and check what your Pharmaceutical drugs are mugging from your body. Have a discussion with your doctor about the supplementation you want to take to replace the mugged minerals.
- Chat with your doctor about what you would need to do, and what markers you would need to achieve, to wean off of your Pharmaceutical drugs.
- As you eat organic veggies and fruits, from all colors of the rainbow, your body will start to heal itself.

What's in your Medicine Box?

Before I got autoimmune disease, I was under the assumption that things I bought over the counter couldn't hurt me.

Boy was a surprised to discover this is not true.

Let's start with the most common drugs we take daily, and let me explain my findings. Understand that this is what I chose to believe and do after researching. Since I am not a scientist and only a concerned citizen that got very sick with inflammation and autoimmune disease, I have made a cautionary decision to avoid as many chemicals as possible, in all aspects of my life and that also includes drugs.

There are alternatives that the body will like and function well on. I will explain after I list all of the common painkillers.

Aspirin

You probably already know that Aspirin is very hard on the stomach. In his article *An Aspirin A Day Causes More Harm Than Good,* on his website, Dr. Josh Axe explains[312] "Other than occasional use, aspirin could be problematic for any of the following conditions.

1. "Heart failure
2. "Asthma
3. "Stomach ulcers
4. "Bleeding or clotting disorders
5. "Diabetes (the American Diabetes Association advises people with diabetes take only the very lowest dosage of aspirin)"

An Article in <u>Mayo Clinic</u> website on the Heart called *Can you take aspirin if you regularly take ibuprofen or another nonsteroidal anti-inflammatory drug (NSAID) for another condition?*[313]

"Side effects and complications of taking aspirin include:[314]

- **"Stroke caused by a burst blood vessel** – While daily aspirin can help prevent a clot-related stroke, it may increase your risk of a bleeding stroke (hemorrhagic stroke).
- **"Gastrointestinal bleeding** – Daily aspirin use increases your risk of developing a stomach ulcer. And, if you have a bleeding ulcer or bleeding anywhere else in your gastrointestinal tract, taking aspirin will cause it to bleed more, perhaps to a life-threatening extent.
- **"Allergic reaction** – If you're allergic to aspirin, taking any amount of aspirin can trigger a severe allergic reaction."

Additional side effects from Dr. Josh Axe[315] – "Again, when there is more than occasional use[316]

- "Kidney failure
- "Liver failure
- "Ulcers – Aspirin is the second leading cause of ulcers
- "Tinnitus

- "Hemorrhagic stroke
- "Reye's syndrome – Aspirin can be fatal for children."

Advil and Aleve – NSAIDS[317]

Very similar to Aspirin, NSAIDS may increase the risk of heart attacks and strokes. They can cause ulcers. They can cause gastrointestinal bleeding. If you have any of the following conditions, there is a greater risk of complication:

- High Blood Pressure
- Fluid retention
- Kidney disease
- Liver disease
- Anemia
- Asthma
- Nasal congestion
- Stomach ulcer
- IBD, Inflammatory bowel disease

I think one of the most important things for you to consider is how hard these drugs are on your gut. Since the goal is to heal leaky gut, eliminating these drugs is a significant step in you healing your inflammation.

Tylenol – Acetaminophen

In addition to plain Tylenol, many over the counter drugs have Acetaminophen in them, so each of these items that you ingest together increases your risk for complication.

Acetaminophen is responsible for 56,000 visits to the emergency room alone and is responsible for 460 deaths a year.

Beyond those statistics, Acetaminophen is very hard on the liver, much harder than we were initially told. It is toxic to the liver, and long-term consumption has detrimental effects to the liver.[318]

It depletes the body of glutathione, which is not only critical to the function of the liver but crucial in healing leaky gut. Taking Acetaminophen with alcohol causes kidney damage.

I was allergic to aspirin since I was little, so Tylenol was my over the counter drug of choice. Although I stayed within the limits for dosage on the bottle, when I was a young adult, I often took Tylenol when I was drinking. I also often took Tylenol daily, for the flu, a headache, any little hiccup that caused pain. No wonder my liver tests are slightly off now, exasperated by the fact that I had serious Mono in my 20's that caused jaundice.

CONCLUSION ON OVER THE COUNTER PAIN KILLERS

They are not good for your body, so try and avoid them. I just listened to a seminar that stated that Aspirin and NSAIDS are the 15th leading killer in America. (Dr. Josh Axe. *Chronic Pain Relief: 14 All-Natural Painkillers* February 24, 2017)

WHAT TO DO INSTEAD?

- **CURCUMIN**

My go-to remedy is Curcumin with black pepper; I use the one from Nature's Sunshine. The Black pepper helps the body to assimilate the spice. I take two twice a day for inflammation, but if I have a headache, or any other symptom where I would have taken Tylenol, I take two more Curcumin. Curcumin is an anti-inflammatory, so your body likes it. Also, Curcumin with black pepper (to help the body assimilate the curcumin) has been proven in test results to work as an anti-depressant, and also reduces anxiety.[319]

Curcumin aids against cancer. It helps against heart disease; it aids against Alzheimer's disease.[320]

Other recommendations

- **GINGER**[321] – reduces muscle pain, soothes an upset stomach, reduces inflammation in joints and eases arthritis, it fights infections, it's antioxid*ants* fight Alzheimer's disease, it aids against cancer, it lowers cholesterol, reduces menstrual cramps, and like aspirin, it can thin the blood[322] (In other words, don't take ginger with other blood thinners, be they aspirin or other pharmaceutical's.)

- **OMEGA-3 FATTY ACIDS** – found in a 2006 study to be as effective as ibuprofen in reducing arthritis pain[323]
- The inclusion of more organic fruits and vegetables increases the amount of salicylic acid in your blood (aspirin is acetyl-salicylic acid) making the body naturally more resistant to pain, without the side effects.[324]

You might also want to check out this article on the top 10 drugs that cause damage to your kidneys. From **Home Gardening Future** in an article from Sept 26, 2016, called *Top 10 Drugs That Cause Kidney Damage* they list even more drugs that impact kidney health.

ANTIBIOTICS

There is no doubt that Antibiotics have tremendous benefits for our body to fight an infectious disease or a bacterial infection.

But, they are useless against viral infections; and still, people take them for viral infections anyway.

The overuse of antibiotics has caused the new Superbugs, which are resistant to known antibiotics. (This is exasperated by the use of antibiotics in our industrial meat and fish industries and is becoming a problem of epic proportions.) (See my Part 3, Chapter 14, **Factory farmed meat, chicken and fish and good alternatives**)

Suzy Cohen RPh, Functional Medicine practitioner and Registered Pharmacist, continues in her blog *Antibiotics Are Stupid – It's Up To You To Be Smart* March 19, 2012:

"Short term effects of antibiotic use include indigestion, stomach pain, gas, nausea, constipation and irritable bowel symptoms and possibly Clostridia difficile, a dangerous infection that causes prolonged watery diarrhea, incredible muscle weakness and fatigue and massive nutrient depletions.[325] Long-term suppression of probiotics often leads to weight gain, yeast overgrowth, vaginal yeast infections, skin problems, chronic fatigue, body aches (fibromyalgia), joint pain, immune suppression and a terribly leaky gut (which then promotes sudden food sensitivities to wheat, dairy and other foods), leading to inflammation.[326]

"The biggest negative about taking Antibiotics, however, is that they don't discriminate. They kill the bad bacteria, but they also kill the good bacteria in your gut. We know how important it is to have a healthy gut with lots of good bacteria to fight leaky gut and inflammation.

"Antibiotics are stupid; they can't distinguish bad bacteria from good ones which mean your camp of friendly flora or 'probiotics' is destroyed. So, to answer your question about long-term side effects, they are tied to the potent drug mugging effect, meaning antibiotic drugs literally 'mug' you of your probiotics. Low probiotics mean low production of methylcobalamin (B-12), vitamin K-2, biotin or folate."[327]

Natural remedies to try first —

Please discuss all changes to your health regimen with your doctor, since I am not one:

"Oregano — It's a strong anti-fungal and may be useful for Candida, as well as parasites. Some people dilute it with a little coconut oil and apply it to the skin (not on broken skin, though), where there are signs of fungal infection. The caracole component of wild oregano oil has activity against MRSA and C. difficile. This may be good for gastrointestinal infections. The taste is pungent you will likely want to dilute this or take a commercial preparation. Carvacrol and thymol are the active ingredients, and this can also help with psoriasis, bladder infections, sinusitis, warts, food poisoning, gum disease and bad breath. If you go to pubmed.com and put in 'carvacrol' or 'thymol' you will see a lot of research done on the active constituent of oregano oil (and thyme which provides thymol).

"Manuka honey — May be helpful on skin infections and gut infections. Raw organic honey is golden when it comes to infections, and research on this particular brand 'Manuka' suggests it kills a wide variety of organisms among them, but that doesn't mean other types of raw (unfiltered) organic golden aren't good:"[328]

CONCLUSION ON ANTIBIOTICS

There are times when we need them. When I got a wild pack of bad bacteria in my gut (from drinking a probiotic drink from an organic farm that was contaminated), the natural remedies above just wouldn't put a dent into what was bad growing in my gut. And all of those little buggers were resistant to regular antibiotics, so I had to take a super antibiotic. However, it did kill off everything, and then I had to start with prebiotics and probiotics to "replant" the good guys back in my gut. After taking the antibiotic, I had diarrhea for weeks. I am finally back to normal taking prebiotic and probiotic supplements.

Prebiotics and Probiotics are important to take every day to make sure you have plenty of good bacteria in your gut.

- For probiotics, you can eat plain yogurt and kefir. You can also eat fermented foods and drink Kombucha.
- For prebiotics, you can eat foods like jicama, onions, garlic, leeks, rye, chicory, blueberries, bananas, asparagus, and artichokes.
- Prebiotics are important because they feed the probiotics in your gut.
- There are also good prebiotics and probiotic supplements to take. I take Klare. I also take Klare enzymes so that I maximize the good nutrients going through my gut wall.

INFLAMMATION

I take Curcumin BP, Quercetin, and Resveratol and up the quantity. These are anti-inflammatory and douse the flame. I use a magnesium spray on my aches and pains. Relaxes unhappy muscles. I avoid any of my triggers.

COLD REMEDIES

Since I no longer take all of the things above, what do I do when I get a cold?[329] Just as a note, while I am writing this, I have a cold. It started yesterday and using the items below; I am already feeling better and probably 50% through the cold, so for me, this works.

I found these suggestions in a blog by functional MD Aviva Romm called *How 7 Top Herbalists and Doctors Fight the* **Flu** *7/22/2013*[330]*:* (she is a Yale trained MD, and Herbalist and a Mid-wife)

- Echinacea Goldenseal
- *Oscillococcinum*
- *Immunocare II* by Natura

- *FLEW AWAY* by Natura
- *Freeze Dried Stinging Nettles*
- *Sambucol,* which is elderberry

I have also had personal success with the following:

SORE OR SCRATCHY THROAT

- ***Mickelberry Elderberry Tonic with Honey***
- ***Mickelberry Elderberry Throat and Lung Tonic***

ANOTHER GREAT THROAT SPRAY

- **Vitality Works** Throat Ease

Dr. Tieraona Low Dog just noted in her Facebook posting Dec 26, 2016, that a new study showed that Elderberry and Echinacea used in combination, are as effective as Tamiflu. Keep these items on hand. These items are important to use immediately when you feel the symptoms of a cold or flu coming on. I have used Echinacea Goldenseal for years, and have added the Sambucol (Elderberry) recently. It works for me.

Cough drops

- ZAND Herbalozenge Lozenges, Orange C, Natural Orange Flavor (sweetened with brown rice syrup)

HAY-FEVER

Some of the major side effects of antihistamines

- Dry mouth
- Drowsiness
- Dizziness
- Nausea and vomiting
- Restlessness or moodiness (in some children)
- Trouble peeing or not being able to pee
- Blurred vision
- Confusion

And for me the drowsiness was horrific. It didn't matter if I tried **Claritin** or **Allegra**. I couldn't stay awake. I ended up taking **Benadryl**, which was known to cause drowsiness but didn't seem to for me. I was taking two every morning, and two every night. Then I read an article that it is believed that **Benadryl** may cause Alzheimer's. Yikes! So, I started looking for a natural substitute.[331]

NATURAL REMEDIES FOR HAYFEVER[332]

- For hay-fever, I use <u>Quercetin</u> (I was using **Benadryl** 2 in the AM and 2 in the PM, and get the same relief from Quercetin without the potential health issues down the line from **Benadryl**.) **Quercetin** is an antioxidant, so your body will love it anyway. Can be taken long term so that you build up resistance when hay fever season begins.
- I also buy local honey at our farmers' market and have a small taste every day. This seems to help me build up some defense against local pollens.
- Stinging Nettle

From Dr. Axe[333] in his blog post 5 Proven, Remarkable Stinging Nettle Benefits

"Stinging nettle has a rich history of medicinal use dating back to medieval Europe where it was used as a diuretic to relieve people of joint pain. According to the University of Maryland Medical Center, studies suggest that it can effectively treat a wide range of health concerns including:

- "Urinary problems like urinary tract infections
- "Benign prostatic hyperplasia
- "Hay fever (allergic rhinitis)
- "Joint pain and strains
- "Insect bites"

CONSTIPATION

I love this one. It shouldn't have been such a surprise to me. After all, as a child, I used Phillips Milk of Magnesia when necessary. Now, instead, I take 2 Magnesium pills (I buy from Suzy Cohen's supplement line.) I am regular as clockwork. The only thing that happens if you take too much magnesium is you get a little loose, so then I back off to 1 at night. Works like a charm.

We have depleted our magnesium in the soil that we are growing our food in. Magnesium, like Vitamin D, is something that most of us are deficient in. The magnesium you are taking above is necessary for hundreds of chemical reactions in the body. Taking it daily is all good!

ACID BLOCKERS

According to Suzy Cohen, in her article *New Study – Suppressing Acid 24/7 Raises Risk of Stroke* 12/1/2016

"The sheer mechanism of action of antacids and acid-blocking drugs will negatively impact your microbiomes (probiotic status) which over time, leads to a reduction in neurotransmitters which are needed for sleep, self-esteem, appetite, mood stability, happiness, and passion. That may sound weird to you, but there are more neurotransmitters a.k.a. 'happy brain chemicals' in your gastrointestinal tract than in your brain. So, a reduction in those probiotics means there will be a 'reduction' in mood as far as I'm concerned.

"All these happy brain chemicals go kaput over time when you lose neurotransmitter balance. Balance is essential. You may over time develop anxiety, phobias of all sorts, anhedonia, agoraphobia and insomnia, nightmares, greater pain and dozens of other neurological symptoms that are hard to pin down to medication because they develop over time. These symptoms can develop from the chronic intake of dozens of different medications that affect your probiotic status, and antibiotics would be the worst of all because those cause severe microbiome shifts."[334]

In other words, don't take them. Ever! Not the over the counter variety. Not the prescription variety. In addition, they increase your risk of food sensitivities and sudden food allergies.

Instead, clean up what you are eating and reduce the discomfort. That's as good a reason as there is to go green. (Lots of healthy organic green vegetables)

Suzy recommends the following if you have continual gastric upset:[335]

- GI-friendly herbs
- Demulcents (marshmallow, slippery elm)
- Herbal teas
- Calendula or chamomile herbal extracts or teas
- Probiotic strains that are natural to your own flora fingerprint, especially lactic acid bacteria and bifido strains.
- Gentle exercise
- Diet restrictions – Pay attention to what foods you eat when the upset begins. For me, it was tomato products and orange juice
- Stress-reducing and joy-provoking activities
- Alcohol and nicotine restriction

Suzy recommends the following remedy if you are suffering from gastric upset, in her article *5 Minute Health Hacks*, 12/12/2016[336]

"**Heartburn** – So, you ate the whole foot-long with chili? Shame on you, now reflux is going to haunt you all night, and probably tomorrow, lol! Try putting a half teaspoon of baking soda in a glass of water, and sip it. Some experts suggest more, but I like to use the lowest effective dose. Make sure this trick is fine with your doctor because it increases the pH in your gut (it's the opposite of an acid blocker). It should help on contact."

PETROLEUM JELLY

How many items in our Medicine chest are made with Petroleum Jelly? Have you ever thought about where it originates? As per the name, it comes from the gas and oil industry. From Vaseline to Vicks VapoRub to Neosporin, the base is petroleum jelly.

"There are side effects and dangers of this ingredient as well. The most frightening thing is that these products may be carrying carcinogenic or cancer causing ingredients. These ingredients get attached to the petroleum jelly during manufacture. Neither the raw material nor the final products are checked for harmful ingredients."[337]

The EWG says "and governments and the CCTFA acknowledge 'there is a risk of contamination from polycyclic aromatic hydrocarbons (PAHs), cancer-causing chemicals found in crude oil and its by-products. While no studies have ever shown a direct link between petrolatum and cancer, the European Union put numerous grades of petrolatum on a list of dangerous substances. Only highly refined petroleum jelly can be used in cosmetics in the EU'.[338]

"The results on the skin from using petroleum jelly are deceiving. While dry skin may feel better when petroleum jelly is applied, it actually is having an adverse effect. The petroleum jelly coats the skin, allowing the chemicals from it to absorb. At the same time, it doesn't enable the body to secrete what it needs to get rid of through sweat. So, while it may feel good, petroleum jelly traps in toxins while offering up some of its own as well. Pretty impressive stuff, right?"[339]

ALTERNATIVES to Petroleum Jelly

So, what have I found that I use and I recommend to you? Products made with avocado oil from **Keys Soaps.**

- *AvoJel*
- *Heat Cool*
- *Urban Shield*
- *Vapor Jell*
- *Zinc Care*
- *Feet and Hand* – alternative Goldbond for dry cracking skin
- *Skin-Aid* – alternative to Bactine
- *Urban Shield* – alternative to Triple Neem oil

FOR INGROWN TOENAILS, OR SKIN FUNGUS

- **Super PAV**[340]

I have had a problem with ingrown toenails for years, and it ends up that yeast on my toes makes the skin grow under the nail. Super PAV has done the trick. I used to buy the one in petroleum jelly, but now am using the straight oil sparingly. Problem solved. This also cured the cracked skin on my heels. Amazing. (I had what I called retailers feet from my years of standing on my feet in retail management. My feet also stunk and if I took off my shoes, I could clear a 1 block radius. Remember the ad where the woman takes off her shoes and the dog plays dead? That was me. Ha! All gone now.)

MUSCLE PAIN

- First of all, I use a topical magnesium spray that relaxes the muscles and works like a charm.
- Activation Products, Ease Magnesium Spray[341]

Second, I use essential oils in a coconut oil base for muscle and joint pain. My favorites are Frankincense and Helichrysum Italicum, but they are quite expensive, so I also use a succotash of other oils that are all good for muscle and joint issues. I am sensitive to the mint family, but if you are not, these are great oils to add to your cream. I use the brand **Rocky Mountain**[342], but you may have a different company that you like. Just make sure you are using oils that are not synthetics.

INSECT REPELLANT

- *DEET* is an insecticide. "Combined exposure to DEET and permethrin, a mosquito spray ingredient, can lead to motor deficits and learning and memory dysfunction."[343]

I have two solutions –

- TEA TREE OIL and LAVENDER OIL COMBINATION

I discovered this years ago on a trip to India. If you put a little of this oil on a moist washcloth and apply it to uncovered skin, the bugs stay away. It works like magic. However, I will warn you; it doesn't smell good.

Some years ago, I was traveling with my female business partner, and we had to go through Calcutta on our way to Bangkok, with a layover. We were in the airline executive waiting room, and as I sat on the upholstered sofa, something bit me. I pulled out my tea tree oil and put it all over my body. My partner went "ewww", and said she would not use it because of the smell. By the time we got to Bangkok, I had only one insect bite, but my partner was covered with large bites all over her body and ended up at a hospital. Tea tree oil works.

The lavender is also an insect deterrent, and it helps the smell, but you can still smell the strong odor of tea tree oil. Use it anyway.

Recently I found a new bug repellant **ForceX** by **Keys-Soaps**. It is a winner. It not only repels bugs, it also sooths an existing bug bite.

Hand sanitizers

I never liked to use them, except when I was in a foreign country. Ends up, many of these are not good for you at all. There are products that are hand sanitizers listed on the EWG site, so search for Hand Sanitizers EWG and see if your product is on the safe list. The best solution is hot water and soap. No matter if you are using a Sanitizer product or soap and water, it is important that you rub your hands together 20 times or more get under your fingernails and between your fingers so that you eradicate all the bacteria. The FDA requested a list of ingredients from companies selling these products, and we should see the results of their research sometime this year (2017).

Finally, pharmaceutical drugs – I suggest you discuss with your doctor that long term, you want to limit your use of Pharmaceutical drugs. Come up with a plan together so that if possible, you can get healthy enough to go off your medications. Eating clean for a while, with lots of organic veggies from all colors of the rainbow, should give your body the nutrients it needs to start to heal itself. Set what the markers would be to start to wean off the pills. And then set your mind to accomplish those goals. Only do this in partnership with your doctor. He overrides any decision you make to get off heavy Pharmaceuticals.

I also suggest that you pick up a copy of Suzy Cohen's **Drug Muggers** Rodale Books; (February 15, 2011). Many of the drugs that we take mug other nutrients from our bodies that we need, so taking a supplement with them might be in order. I certainly was surprised to discover what deficiencies I had as a result of the Pharmaceutical medications I was on. It's worth owning the book and referring to it for your health.

I am not a MD, so any of my suggestions are what has worked for me. You may want to consult with your physician for further guidance. (And as discussed in Part 1 of this book, I recommend that that MD is a Functional MD, if at all possible.)

Chapter 19

Cleaning Supplies

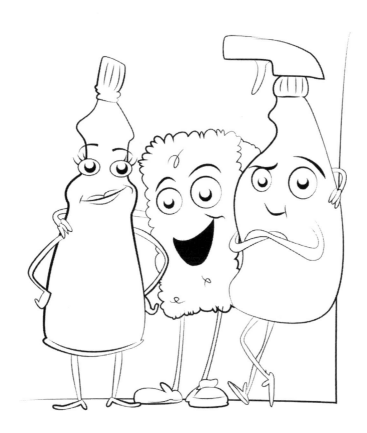

Dousing the flame of inflammation:

THE BIG TAKEAWAYS ON CLEANING SUPPLIES

- Many, if not most, of the ingredients in your cleaning supplies are toxic.
- Toxic ingredients cause leaky gut, and create pain.
- Look up what you are using on the Environmental Working Group site, and see just how toxic they are.
- Choose items that are rated either an A or a B.
- Many of the ingredients in your cleaning products also pose environmental risks.

By now, it is probably no surprise to you if you have read the previous chapters in this book. Your cleaning supplies are loaded with toxins.

I read, not long ago, that the most toxic substance in your home was your detergent. Both the detergent to wash your clothes and the detergent to wash your dishes are most likely horrifically toxic. So, toxic that if your toddler ate one of those cute little pods, he would probably die before you could get him to the emergency room.

Wow, isn't that frightening?

EWG published their *EWG'S Guide to Health Cleaning* in 2012 and recently analyzed thousands of product labels and images and hundreds of company websites to update their guide in 2016.

"Although consumers increasingly are making purchasing decisions based on safety and transparency, no federal or state laws have been implemented that require disclosure of cleaning products' ingredients – not on the label nor online." There are huge areas of concern, and at least now we have the **EWG** database with information on 2500 products to use as a guide in choosing the safest products for your home.[345]

Companies have made it very difficult for consumers to know what was in them. "These products commonly contain chemicals that can cause reproductive problems, exacerbate asthma, burn or irritate your skin and harm the environment. Some have even been linked to cancer.[346]

The Guide now contains information on more than 2,500 products, letting you easily learn about the health hazards and ecological concerns associated with the thousands of chemicals in cleaners. It's meant to help you make smarter, healthier choices, which will continue to push the cleaners market toward greater safety and transparency. Ratings range from A to F.

In 2016 "**EWG** added or updated information for 406 products from 85 brands. They focused on the products you use most frequently – laundry (188 products), dish (124) and all-purpose (94) cleaners. The products highlighted were found on store shelves from October 2015 to February 2016 or were submitted directly to **EWG** by manufacturers. In addition to product packaging, labels, and websites, information came from ingredient disclosure documents and worker safety data sheets, required by the **U.S. Occupational Safety and Health Administration.**"[347]

Highlights of the report:[348]

- Only 1 in 7 got an A or a B because of the toxic ingredients in them
- More than 25% of the products had ingredients in them that are carcinogenic.
- 20% of the products had ingredients that had developmental, endocrine or reproductive issues.
- 70% of the products listed "fragrance" which most likely are endocrine disrupters.
- Only 14% got full credit for disclosing ingredients on the label, and another 14% for disclosure on product websites.
- 10% of the products were corrosive and could cause damage to skin and eyes.
- 10% of products had substances that cause skin allergies and a high possibility of skin damage.
- 60% had ingredients that posed environmental risks. "These chemicals are only partly removed by wastewater treatment plants, don't readily break down, are persistent in the environment and toxic to aquatic life."
- Fewer than 40% were rated "good" for disclosing information about ingredients in their products.

I could go on, but you get the picture. There is no regulation; there is only partial disclosure, and these products are poisoning us and our environment.

So, what do we do?

Throw all the crappy cleaners in your house into the dumpster. You might want to check with your waste disposal company first, to make sure they don't have special rules to accept toxic chemicals, but if they do, they will give you instructions as to what to do with these toxic cleaners.

What do I use?

I found an amazing cleaner two years ago that was made with plant enzymes. At first, my cleaning lady thought I was nuts that this one product was going to clean my dishes, my windows, my sinks and counters, my floors, my shower stall but after trying it for a couple of weeks, she became a believer. I love this product. It is called **BRANCH BASICS.**

Well, last year they discovered it had an ingredient in it that was a synthetic, so they immediately removed their product and informed all of their users. The good news is that they have now reformulated, and the new product is due to be reintroduced soon.

What I love about this company is that they are committed to their mission. Their product wasn't what they thought it was. It wasn't up to their standards. So, no questions asked; they simply removed it from the market, even though they had no reports of any issues with their product.

When it comes back on the market, I strongly recommend that you give it a try. The relaunch is scheduled for Summer 2017

To share with you how amazing I think this product is, I always hated making eggs, because whether they were poached, scrambled or fried, the residue stuck to the bottom of the pan and was hard to remove. Well, soak it a minute in a little **Branch Basics,** and it slides right off.

Until I found a shampoo that wasn't making my head itchy (and I now use **Key-Soaps** shampoo) I was even washing my hair with **Branch Basics**. And my hair looked great!

Branch Basics is so clean, one night I mistakenly used it in lieu of vinegar in a salad dressing. We ate quite a bit of salad before I missed the "tang" of the vinegar.

Neither my husband nor I had any ill effects from ingesting the cleaner. (I am more careful now. Ha!)

Unfortunately, with Branch Basics unavailable for the last year, I had to find alternate products. All of these are listed to be an A on the EWG scale.

Many of these products are from Seventh Generation which gave EWG full disclosure.

Toilet Bowl Cleaner

- Seventh Generation Toilet Bowl Natural Cleaner, Emerald Cypress and Fir – Rating A

Dishwasher Detergent Packs

- Seventh Generation Dishwasher Packs, Free and Clear – Rating A

Dishwashing Liquid

- Sun and Earth Dishwashing Liquid Extra Concentrated, Light Citrus – Rating A

Cleanser

Cleanser for sink and tubs

- ***Bon Ami*** (what my mother used to use back in the 50's and 60's) I bought it from ***Thrive Markets*** – Rating A

Mold Control

- Concrobium – Rating A

I just read that Tea Tree Oil and Lavender are also great for Mildew. I am going to try that out. I have a little on the outside of my shower door and on the rim in my washing machine.

I recently read that tea tree oil works wonders on mold. Will give it a shot.

Hydrogen Peroxide is also supposed to be good.

Detergent

- Planet 2 Ultra Laundry Detergent, Free & Clear – Rating A
- Seventh Generation Natural Laundry Detergent Powder, Free and Clear – Rating A

Bleach

- Seventh Generation Chlorine-Free Bleach, Free and Clear – Rating A

Floor Cleaning, Tile cleaning, etc. I am still using my Branch Basics

I no longer use any wax to polish my wood floors or my wood furniture. I use Branch Basics to wash my windows and my linoleum. When the new product comes out, I will use it for many of the tasks above.

OTHER SUGGESTIONS

- HEPA filter vacuum
- An air filter in each room you live in. The air inside your home could be more toxic than the air outside.
- Change furnace and air conditioning filters at least yearly.
- Do a test on your home for **mold**. It can be expensive, but mold mimics many autoimmune symptoms, so it's well worth the expense. It could save your life. If your home has mold, there is also a rather expensive test to detect mold in your body. 25% of the population is bothered by mold. I happen to be one of them. But thank goodness, my home tested mold free.
- Check online for Radon to see if the area where you live have issues. If so, test for **Radon gas**.

For more information on mold see http://www.survivingmold.com/diagnosis.

Chapter 20

Toxic Metals

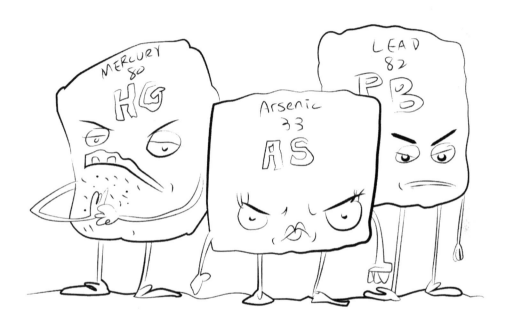

Dousing the flame of inflammation:

THE BIG TAKEAWAYS ON TOXIC METALS

- From Natural News: "According to the United States Environmental Protection Agency, the average American has over 700 chemicals in his or her body — a terrible toxic burden, and one our bodies are ill-equipped to handle. Exposure to toxic chemicals and heavy metals is occurring at a level unprecedented in human history — triggering the development of devastating illnesses such as Alzheimer's disease, diabetes, autoimmune disease, and cancer."
- Get rid of your mercury amalgams. Find a biological dentist in your area. Your dentist will probably not understand this and isn't equipped to do the procedure. But the first step is to eliminate one of the main sources of your poisoning.
- You have to make sure to nourish your body with a lot of yummy nutrients and minerals before you can begin to detox.
- You need to test to make sure you can methylate. Otherwise, the metals will come out and go right back into to your fat and your bones where they hide.
- I am on stage 2 of releasing the metals from my body. I have my fingers crossed that this will work, but there is a stage 3 if needed.

Let me start by telling you my story.

I was born in 1949 in Pittsburgh, PA. I popped out allergic to Pittsburgh. I was named Miss Mess by my doctor and had weekly allergy shots from as far back as I can remember. (This was an event for me because, after each shot, the Doctor gave me a bag of little candy hearts for being a brave little girl. At 3, I wanted to marry him. Ha!)

I do remember trucks oiling the street in front of our house near Pittsburgh to keep the coal and steel dust down.

My parents moved me to California when I was 5, to improve my health. Moving to California certainly helped. I was much healthier than I had been in Pittsburgh.

When we went back to visit family, (by car), I would break out in hives about 25 miles out of the Pittsburgh general area. I was truly allergic or sensitive to Pittsburgh.

Flash forward to 2 years ago. In doing research, I came upon an explanation that metal toxicity was one of the contributors to inflammation, and ultimately to autoimmune disease. Both of my parents had died of diseases that looked as if they could have been exasperated by the toxins in the air in Pittsburgh. (It seems to be generally cleaned up now, by the way.) So, I wanted to be tested.

During my first appointment with my brand new functional MD, I asked to be tested. My functional doctor was amused by my story and agreed to test me.

Walla, I was loaded with them. I had excess mercury, lead, cadmium, arsenic, nickel, copper, zinc, antimony and thallium. I hit the Mother Lode!

I want to share this with you, because if you have cleaned up your food, and you are eating organic; If you have started eliminating other toxins from your life and your environment; if you have done the sensitivity tests, and eliminated the problematic foods; this might be your next key to wellness. It is worth investigating.

Finding that I had all of these toxic metals in my body also is an explanation of why it has been so difficult for me to lose weight. So, I kind of felt "Eureka," I might actually get to the bottom of my health issues.

However, learning this ended up just taking another layer off the onion of my body dysfunction.

The first question my Functional MD asked me, after reviewing my metal load, was an interesting one. Had I noticed that my body over-reacted to over the counter medications in my past?

Well, yes indeed, I had always known that. If for example, I needed Phillips Milk of Magnesia, the instructions might be to take 2, and I would take ½. Otherwise, my body would immediately go in the opposite direction, and that became a whole new problem. This was true for me with many over the counter medicines.

It ends up; we tested to see if I had a Methylation problem. Methylation is a relatively new test, and it measured if I have any DNA anomalies regarding this important body function, and bingo, I did indeed.

What this meant is that my body couldn't readily detoxify. I know I don't sweat like normal people, but my entire detoxification system is hindered by these markers that I inherited from one or both of my parents. Geeze. I wish I had known this to help them when they were alive and had gotten terribly ill.

So, we started on a year program to improve my detoxification functions before we could even consider detoxing the Heavy Metals.

We started with a liver detox. That lasted several months. I actually did the liver cleanse twice to get improved liver function. I then had an appointment to go weekly for what was called an intravenous "Meyer's Cocktail" to beef up vitamins that were deficient in my body, like B-12 and Vitamin C and magnesium. It also had glutathione, which helped my liver repair, all in preparation for the heavy metal detox to come.

I added Milk Thistle to my supplements, again for my liver.

We added L-5 MTHF to my supplement routine, and also SAMe. (I take a lot of L-5 MTHF). Then we added NAC and DIM.

It was important for me to improve my ability to detox. The toxic metals hide in fat and our bones. If I pulled them out of their hiding places, and if my body couldn't handle removing them from my system, they would simply recirculate right back into their hiding places.

I found a biological dentist and had my amalgams removed.

Just a note, I love my 80-year-old dentist, and I think he is terrific, but he thought I lost my mind with this. So, if you share what you are doing with anyone in conventional medicine, (MD or Dentist) they are bound to scratch their head in disbelief. Do it anyway. (It made sense to me that I didn't want the mercury toxin in my body.)

It is really important that you go to a dentist that protects you and his office in the process of getting these removed. When you have them removed, it is a scene from a science fiction movie, they wear masks and breathe oxygen; you have on a mask. They cover their heads and their faces. They use special suction equipment, and they also suck it out of the air. The mercury amalgams are removed without you ingesting the toxic material. Win!

I started this process in January 2015. In August 2016, my Functional MD thought I was ready to start to detox. And we took aim at mercury. I took **MetalloClear** by **Metagenic**s. (Do not try this alone. Do this with a functional practitioner for every step of the process.)

In November 2016, I was tested again for toxic metals. The mercury was gone. YIPPEE! Small victory. However, although the other toxic metals were definitely diminished from all of the work we had done, they were still present in toxic quantities.

In January 2017, I started on the next leg of my detox journey. I am taking a chlorella drop, herbal detox. I increase the drops every two days. In the beginning, I got headaches and a stomach ache, but that is less annoying as I build up a tolerance. I did this throughout the months of January and February. I will remain at the high dosage through March and April. I am experiencing "flares" as the toxins come out of hiding. In May, we will test again.

If this round of detoxifying doesn't do it, there is yet another way to detox that will be even harder on my body, but that should do the trick. I feel like the Terminator; I want them out. *smile*.

In an article called ***Heavy metals alert – How to safely detoxify the body*** [350] by Jonathon Landsman with Wendy Myers, November 10, 2016, in **Natural News** on the web, it states:

"According to the United States Environmental Protection Agency, the average American has over 700 chemicals in his or her body – a terrible toxic burden, and one our bodies are ill-equipped to handle. Exposure to toxic chemicals and heavy metals is occurring at a level unprecedented in human history — triggering the development of devastating illnesses such as Alzheimer's disease, diabetes, autoimmune disease, and cancer."

We know it has been noted as a problem with leaky gut and autoimmune disease, and that they cause inflammation. Each metal has its own repertoire of problems. Toxic metals are everywhere, and impossible to avoid, so it's highly likely, if you have pain, that you have toxic metals in your system.

So, let's talk about things these nasty metals do to the body. Wendy Myers article *"Guide to Sources and Symptoms of Toxic Metals"* from her website **Live to 110** lists each metal and the harmful effects on our bodies. Her specialty is heavy toxic metals. The impact on the body of the different toxic metals is staggering.

The following list, from Dr. Joseph Mercola, ND, in an article called *"Toxic Metals: They Reason You Still Feel Sick"* July 22, 2008, on his website,[351] shows the wide range of complications:

- Sudden, severe cramping and convulsions
- Nausea
- Vomiting
- Sweating
- Headache
- Difficulty breathing
- Impaired cognitive, motor and language skills
- Fatigue
- Digestive distress, and reduced ability to properly assimilate and utilize fats
- Aching joints
- Depression
- Impaired blood sugar regulation
- Female reproductive problems such as menstrual difficulties, infertility, miscarriage, pre-eclampsia, pregnancy-induced hypertension and premature birth

Dr. Mercola then notes in the same article that "Dr. Kaayla Daniel, and Dr. Galen Knight have observed that even when people follow healthy dietary guidelines, they can still have serious health problems. They may digest their food poorly, experience digestive distress, or be generally sickly."

Dr. Mercola continues: "As Dr. Daniel et.al. explain in this article; optimal nutrition is essential when dealing with metal toxicity because if you are deficient in essential metals, your body will use toxic metals as 'stand-ins' instead. For example:

- "Calcium is replaced by lead, which deposits primarily in bone, and disrupts the formation of red blood cells. Lead contributes to poor bone health such as osteopenia and osteoporosis.
- "Zinc is replaced by cadmium, which tends to accumulate heavily in your kidneys. Cadmium overload is associated with peripheral neuropathy.
- "Magnesium is replaced by aluminum, which, among other things, induces neurochemical changes and has been identified as a contributing factor to developing Alzheimer's.
- "Manganese is replaced by nickel, which is carcinogenic."

Everything you learned in my chapters on Food (Part 3) about how to eat clean and feed your body beautiful nutrients is crucial to your body's ability to purge the metal toxins.

I also now understand why I was given the "Meyers Cocktail" in preparation to the detox.

Once I complete my Heavy Metal Detox, I will write a blog and update how I am doing.

I am still a "health in progress", but I am motivated to do everything and anything I can do to heal my body.

And this is why I can yell out; it feels good to feel good. And I am on a path, to feel even better.

Chapter 21

Toxins in your Kitchen - pots and pans, utensils, and food storage

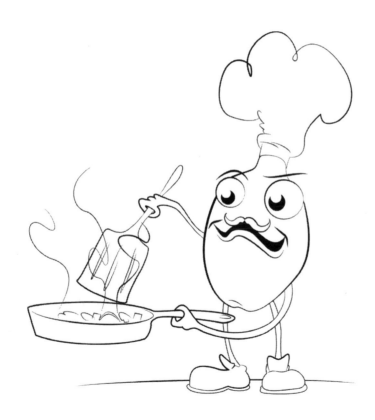

> Dousing the flame of inflammation:
> # THE BIG TAKEAWAYS ON TOXINS IN YOUR KITCHEN
>
> - Teflon is deadly. If you still have Teflon pans in your kitchen, throw them away.
> - Do your research on what alternative pots and pans you can use. Choose something that is safe, that also fits your budget.
> - Food storage is an issue. You must purge all of the plastic out of your kitchen and find an alternative method of storage. It doesn't matter if it is BPA or PET plastic. They are both chemicals that are harmful to the body.
> - I have discovered silicone. I like it. You might want to give it a whirl.
> - Aluminum foil, Saran Wrap and Glad Wrap, all need to be thrown out. In my opinion, it's not worth the risk of the chemicals leaching into your body.
> - Never use plastic of any kind in the microwave. The heat makes the problem worse. Heat causes the chemicals to leach at a greater level.
> - These are my opinions. Research and form your own. My stance is to play it safe. I am committed to removing toxins from my life to reduce inflammation.
> - Plastic cutting boards must go. Wood or bamboo are excellent alternatives.

It's frustrating to discover how toxic many items that I have used in everyday life there really are. I vaguely knew that coated cookware was an issue, but I had a really nice set of pots and pans from a famous maker, and didn't realize that this also referred to these pans.

When I started purging all of the toxins out of my life, I had to take a hard look at what I was using in the kitchen. Like everything, there is disagreement on what is good and what is bad, so we can only do the best that we can do. This is what I have found, and this is how I have solved these issues for myself. Please do some research for yourself and decide what is best for your kitchen.

Pots and Pans

One thing that everyone agrees on, is that Teflon cookware is toxic. Get rid of it, period. I say that now that I have replaced my cookware with stainless steel. But full confession, I have held on to my Teflon fry pan, because it is so very easy to wash. I finally bit the bullet and threw it out.

Let's talk about Teflon first, since I would imagine some of you are as attached to your Teflon cookware like I was. I want you to understand why it is crucial that you give it up. *smile*

Teflon was discovered 70 years ago by DuPont. According to the EPA, they purposely did not disclose that the surface was toxic when they discovered how deadly it was way back in the 1970's. They have been fined over 300 million dollars. They have polluted the communities where their chemicals were manufactured, and destroyed water systems.

Peflourooanoic acid (PFOA), a chemical used to produce Teflon, has been appearing in blood samples of people worldwide.[353]

These chemicals are very difficult to detoxify out of the body. Once it is in your blood, it stays in your blood. EWG released a report that even if you have no additional contact with this chemical, it would take 20 years for the body to detoxify and eliminate it. These chemicals also cause "forever" pollution to our environment. Yikes!

This chemical has been linked to cancer.[354]

The older your pots and pans with Teflon are, the more the chemicals have broken down to deliver a huge hit into your food every time you cook with it.

I guess our first clue should have been when DuPont publicly admitted, that the chemicals used in Teflon killed birds. They still swore there was no danger to humans. Yeah, right!

(Just a side note: unfortunately, pots and pans are not the only place where these chemicals are used. They are also present in stain resistant carpets and flame retardants for clothing and computers; and in nail polishes, eyeglasses and even in the linings of pizza boxes.[355]) It's also on the down side of many of the wrapping papers used in fast food. Yet another reason to NOT EAT FAST FOOD.

Ok, so the Teflon pans go into the dumpster. Now what do we do. This is where the waters get murky and you can find people who have written articles on the subject that point out pros and cons on all the other available materials used in cookware.

Stainless Steel

Most experts consider Stainless Steel to be the best alternative. This is what we chose for our kitchen. Stainless steel is inert, so it does not react with your food. It is more difficult to clean. And we bought a really good set, which is rather heavy, so I also consider that a con. For all my pan types, I really enjoy using my stainless steel. My one exception is my fry pan – I haven't made the leap to enjoying stainless when I need to cook with my fry pan. One tip for making the pan easier to clean: get the pan really hot before you add the food that you are going to cook in the pan. However, I still miss the convenience of my Teflon coated fry pan, so I have been searching for a replacement.

What I decided on was ceramic. I will admit that it does cook like a dream. No more stuck eggs on my pan in the morning, no more hard to clean goop after cooking hamburgers or meats.

Researching for this chapter however, I have discovered that the ceramic that I purchased is only good for about a year. Then it starts to break down and creates its own issues, so I am back to the drawing board.

There is one ceramic brand that seems to be universally loved, and again, it is an expensive choice. Xtrema is recommended by several articles on the best pots and pans available.

Cast Iron

My mother always used cast iron, so I do have a couple of different size fry pans and I do use them fairly often. There seems to be a little disagreement about how much iron you get into your food when using cast iron, and whether or not this is good or bad for you. We need iron, but not in heavy qualities. The biggest downfall, I read, was to be careful cooking with this pan for small children under 3. They don't need the additional iron. The one rule that seems universal is to avoid tomato products in your cast iron skillet – so no more spaghetti sauce or taco meat prepared in this pan. Be sure to keep your cast iron skillet seasoned, which helps lessen how much iron goes into your food.

And alternative to cast iron is ceramic-covered cast iron – These pans are beautiful and expensive. Le Crueset is easy to cook with and clean.

Aluminum Pots and Pans

This is another area where there seems to be disagreement. Since I am in the process of chelating heavy toxic metals out of by body, one of which is aluminum, I would vote that aluminum is not a good choice. Anodized Aluminum seems to be considered acceptable since the manufacturing process locks in the cookware's aluminum content. This anodization does breakdown, however, over time, just like the cast iron, when cooking with acidic foods like tomatoes. However, aluminum does more harm to the body than the iron from cast iron does. Chemical dishwasher soaps can also break down the anodization. (If you follow my recommendations for dishwasher soaps that are not toxic, I would think that might solve this issue.) Cooks like this type of pot because of its anti-stick properties, and ease of cleaning. You decide if this is right for you.

Glass – Pyrex and Corning Ware are safe. I love my Pyrex, especially for baking. I have discovered that Corning Ware is not as unbreakable as the type I had years ago when I first got married. If you can pick up Corning Ware at a garage sale, that is vintage, that would be a win.

I did find one other type of baking pan that I look forward to trying. Stoneware baking pans by **Pampered Chef** were called out on the **Wellness Mama** website.[356] They look great, so I purchased one. **Rada Cutlery** also makes bread pans and other baking shapes and sizes in stoneware.

Utensils for cooking

Ok, the black plastic spatula that I have used and the black plastic spoon that I stirred with is probably not acceptable, so I threw mine away. If they are silicone, you get to keep them. If it's plastic, as you will see when I get to food storage, it's got chemicals in it that you don't want in your body.

I have purchased stainless steel spatulas, slotted spoons, and long forks, and am enjoying them. I also bought two sets of cooking utensils in silicone, and they are great. Love the colors. One set is turquoise, the other is lime green.

Food Storage

Prepare to mortgage your house to replace all of the plastic containers you have been using. (Just joking, sort of.) Finding alternatives to all of the plastic that we are surrounded with was not easy, and in all honesty, there is not an easy solution.

I have food storage sets that are a heavy glass with a BPA-free Bisphenol A plastic lid. (BPA was discussed previously in my book, Chapter 17, **Drinking Water**, as having toxins that leech into our water and foods). I have written to all of the companies that make these to see if the lids are also PET (polyethylene terephthalate) free. No answer yet. PET has recently been discovered to have different issues than the BPA plastics. (Update 2 weeks later, the companies are not calling me back. I finally got through to one person who said she didn't know and seemed unable to check. Not a good sign. I choose to pass.) Previously thought to be safe, EWG recently discovered in testing that PET plastics also leech chemicals that could be harmful to the body.[357] But for now we do the best we can do, and staying away from the BPA is a start.

Just a quick aside, on Amazon, I posted a question to the manufactures about the lids on their glass food storage containers, asking if they were also PET free. Some lovely Amazon customer decided to answer me. "Only suitable for small rodent type PETS. They are not included with container. I hope this helps." I hope he was joking. *smile*

I have also purchased a few silicone container sets. Silicone at this point, is considered safe. The good news is that these containers collapse for easier storage, and have silicone covers. The bad news is that these silicone containers collapse, so they are a little less stable. But being aware of this, I can make them work. These are not inexpensive. But the lids are also silicone, so these are a safe bet.

I just received some silicone bowls with lids that I love. There is a steam release on top if you want to microwave something in them. There is evidence that you should avoid using your microwave. I am not quite ready to give mine up. But never, never microwave food in any kind of plastic. Deadly!

Save your glass jars for future food storage. I also bought a box of Mason jars (Ball jars would also work) which are glass. I am not sure about the plastic rim in the lids, but it's better than an all plastic container.

Stainless steel containers with stainless steel covers are also available for food storage. They would be a good choice. I kind of like to see what I am storing; otherwise the food becomes a science experiment. So, I consider that a con.

Everything seems to come in plastic – so many of our groceries are packaged in plastic. Again, we do the best we can. I even bought bags to put my produce in that are not plastic. Plastic is leaching chemicals into our food and is a major ecological issue. Purifyou Premium Reusable Mesh states that they are manufactured in a factory that is toxic chemical free. However, they do not state what they materials are used. Again. we do the best we can do. These bags can be washed in the clothes washer, which I think is a plus. Again, these are not inexpensive. Update 2 weeks later, they are doing a fine job keeping most of my veggies fresh. Win!

Aluminum foil, wax paper, Saran Wrap, Glad Wrap

These are all toxic....and these are items that I haven't completely figured out how to replace.

Aluminum foil

The FDA doesn't seem to think it is a problem, but then again, look at all the toxins that are allowed in the previous chapters of this book, and decide whether or not you want to believe this. I am loaded with aluminum, and currently trying to detoxify from it, so my decision is "no way".

According to Dr. Joseph Mercola, ND, in an article called **Is It Safe TO Cook With Aluminum Foil** he states "Aluminum has been long known to be neurotoxic, with mounting evidence that chronic exposure is a factor in many neurological diseases, including dementia, autism, and Parkinson's disease."

There are articles that disagree with Dr. Mercola. But note: this is another one of those "absence of evidence" areas when in reality it is an area where there is "evidence of absence." No long-term studies have been done to prove that aluminum is unsafe. Where would the money be in conducting that research?

There is a lot of aluminum in our environment anyway. If the soil that our food is grown in gets acidic, then more aluminum is absorbed by the plants that we eat.

Since all of the chemicals being used to grow food are changing our soil biome, I would bet we are getting a lot of aluminum from our food. I don't need more.

Aluminum is also in antiperspir*ants* and antacids, and I avoid both for a variety of reasons. Antiperspir*ants* were an early allergen (or sensitivity), and I avoid over the counter drugs including antacids, as explained in Chapter 18, **Drugs**.

Again, do your own research and then decide what is best for you.

Wax paper, Saran Wrap and Glad Wrap

You know by now that plastic leaches chemicals that are harmful. Under no circumstances can you microwave food wrapped in these toxic wraps. That makes the problem worse. The question is, once you stop using these products what do you do instead?

The containers I have listed above are your first tool. I was surprised about wax paper. So, what is the wax made of? Petroleum. Ducky. I have already established the negative qualities of Petroleum in products for our body, (see my chapter on Cosmetics, Part 4, Chapter 16), so out it goes.

Bees Wraps are a great solution, but very expensive. It sticks better to itself than to bowls, but is made with wax from bees, and is totally non-toxic, which is a big win. These are pieces of fabric coated in bees wax to wrap over containers for storage. Clever idea. mommypotamus.com also has a recipe to make your own. I am not a handy do-it-yourself kind of gal, but you could make your own less expensive variety, which I think is terrific.[358] These are washable, which is another win.

Parchment Paper

I do use unbleached parchment paper now, in all the pans that I bake in. This really works well and minimizes clean up. (I prefer the unbleached to lessen the chemicals I come into contact with.)

Cutting Boards

If they are plastic, out they go. In addition to leeching chemicals into our food, bacteria gets into the nooks and crannies of the cuts. Not a good look, and not safe.

Wood cutting boards and bamboo cutting boards are the best.

So, how do you clean wood and bamboo cutting boards? I use a double cleaning method of using vinegar[359] and wipe, and then Hydrogen Peroxide[360] (let it sit and fizz, which is what kills the bacteria) and then wipe. I read years ago that these two substances can kill almost any nasty bacteria that might be lurking on your cutting surface. I also clean my kitchen sponges this way, and then I throw it into the dishwasher with my dishes.

As I come up with other solutions, I will update resources on my website, www.cherylmhealthmuse.com

Part 5
Toxic Mindst Toxic Body

Introduction

Toxic Minds

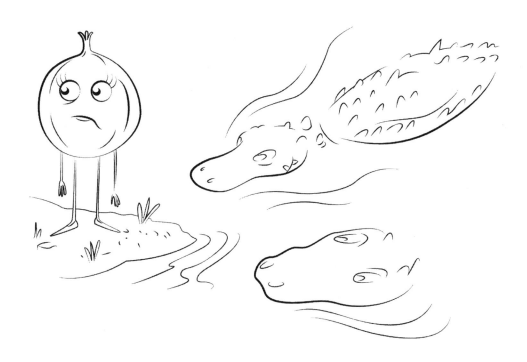

TOXINS IN OUR RELATIONSHIPS, OUR THOUGHTS, AND TOXIC STRESS, AND REMOVING THE TOXIC SLUDGE IN OUR BODIES

THERE IS MORE TO LIFE THAN JUST FOOD. LETS LOOK AT THE OTHER ASPECTS OF LIFE THAT SUSTAIN US –

"In the sweetness of friendship, let there be laughter, and sharing of pleasures, for in the dew of little things the heart finds its morning and is refreshed"

KHALIL GIBRAN

Dousing the flame of inflammation:

THE BIG TAKEAWAYS ON TOXIC MINDS

- There are 12 other primary elements that feed your "heart and soul" and satisfy your hunger for life. These areas are crucial to your wellbeing. Otherwise, you will live without joy and peace, and wellness will be elusive.
- To be healthy, these 12 physical, spiritual and mental primary elements need to be balanced. They are all important.
- Consciously put together a plan to improve any of these areas that are deficient and create a life worth living. Keep working on each of these areas until they are all fulfilling in your life. You deserve to enjoy all 12 elements at their fullest point.
- How you feel about your outer world affects the health of your inner world.
- Cicero – "Diseases of the soul are more dangerous and more numerous than those of the body."
- Mastin Kipp – "It's time to stop operating like everyone's life is more valuable than yours."
- Before you can be a caretaker for others, you must fill your own cup of love.
- Unknown – "Fall in love with taking care of yourself, mind, body and spirit"

These are the 12 primary elements[362] –

266

- Relationships
- Social Life
- Joy
- Spirituality
- Creativity
- Finances
- Career
- Education
- Health
- Physical Activity
- Home Cooking
- Home Environment

Relationships and *Social Life* bring you an opportunity to give and receive love and friendship. They bring community. They also give you love and acceptance.

Spirituality and *Creativity* bring you *Joy*. Spirituality allows you to connect with the universe, something greater than you and gives life its meaning. Creativity allows you freedom of expression, in a way that is uniquely yours.

Finances and *Career* bring you security. In the best-case scenario, Career brings you passion, and Finances reward you for sharing that love with the world.

Education brings you confidence and knowledge. It feeds your dreams and allows you to share with others.

Physical Activity, movement, keeps you flexible, keeps your body humming properly, keeps you healthy, balances your chi, and moves out the toxic sludge of your body.

Home Cooking is critical to eating real food. It was also a significant component of my family life as a child since we all sat around the dinner table and shared our lives. My family had a lot of humor; family stories got retold, and always brought Joy. Home cooking allows you to control what ingredients go into the food that you eat and it allows you to feed your body delicious, high-quality nutrients.

Your *Home Environment* is where you find peace; its space to call your own; it reflects you.

All of these things in balance create **Health**.

How we feel about our outer world impacts how we feel in our inner world.

Happiness and health, at a core level, is the ability to have all 12 of the primary elements at a fulfilling point at the same time.

It is rare for any of us to have all of the 12 primary elements at their most satisfying point. When we are out of balance, we create stress. Stress causes disease. Stress causes inflammation. Stress causes pain.

People with inflammation probably share one thing in common. They haven't been good at taking care of themselves. I was a workaholic, out of balance, and I didn't take care of me. I didn't have all of the aspects of my life in balance. I was a caretaker: for many friends, my family, my staff at work and I was a caretaker for my work. But, I didn't pay attention to myself along the way.

"It's time to stop operating like everyone's life is more valuable than yours."

MASTIN KIPP-*DAILY LOVE*

When I started to pay attention to how I felt, it was a true awakening. I am sure many of you can relate to being a caretaker at the expense of your own well-being and health.

It was when I acknowledged the problem that I began to find solutions and add more joy into my life.

Getting well has to start with taking care of ourselves, filling our own cup, and living with joy. It is when we get out of balance that we also start to get sick. These are the elements of our minds, lives and environment that we need to nourish in order to find joy and happiness. In this part, I am going to address five areas of toxicity:

1. Toxic stress
2. Toxic anxious thoughts
3. Toxic relationships
4. Toxic lack of sleep
5. The toxic effects of a sedentary lifestyle
   - Movement is necessary to remove toxic sludge from detoxification out of your body.
   - Movement gets the blood flowing to bring the healthy nutrients to our organs and our cells.
   - Movement is good for your heart and good for your brain, and essential for your body.
   - Movement releases "happy" hormones.

All five of these areas can suck the life out of us, and until we learn to deal with the stress, calm the toxic thoughts, and eliminate the toxic relationships, get 7-8 hours of sleep consistently, and move, we can't get well.

"Diseases of the soul are more dangerous and more numerous than those of the body"

CICERO

Purging the toxins from these five areas allows us to live with ourselves in happiness and joy.

Health is about all of the things you strive for, but that sometimes seem elusive. It's your epiphany knowing the path forward to the life you deserve.

"When you recover or discover something that nourishes your soul and brings joy, care enough about yourself to make room for it in your life."

JEAN SHINODA BOLEN

I spent much of my life being unhealthy. I lived in fear. I blocked my own happiness. I worked too much. I allowed stress not only to survive but to take permanent residence in my body and my life.

I was stuck in the land that when this, blah, blah, blah, happens, then I can blah, blah, blah. I was never going to be enough. Fear.

So, what happened?

I have jokingly remarked for years that when my angels want me to get a lesson, the first time, they poke me. If I don't get it, the second time, I get a little slap on the face. If I am still not paying attention, I get a big thump on my back. Finally, I get hit with a 2x4.

So, I got a wake-up call.

More accurately I got hit with the big 2x4.

I got sick, really sick.

So, I got out of my own way and found the life I deserved. I became proactive and went out to find it.

I have found the path to wellness. I have found joy and contentment. I became compassionate with myself. Most importantly, I have found love. I have found balance, and although I still have a few challenges to partake in the entire feast, I am well on my way.

If you tackle each area of the 12 primary elements, and revaluate what you can improve and how to do it, and if you give each area the importance it deserves and manifest it in your life, you will find happiness, love, and complete health.

If you are having a difficulty sorting all of this out on your own, again, as a Certified Health Coach, I could help you do it. It's easy to relate to someone who has been through it and has come out the other end.

"Fall in love with taking care of yourself, mind, body and spirit"

UNKNOWN

You deserve to be healthy, loved and happy. We all do!

Remember,

"Eat like you love yourself. Move like you love yourself. Speak like you love yourself. Act like you love yourself."

UNKNOWN

Feast on all of the good things of life.

Chapter 22

Toxic Stress

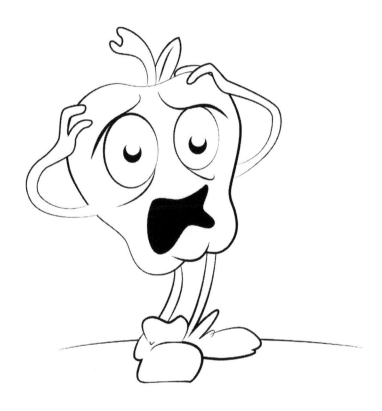

Dousing the flame of inflammation:

THE BIG TAKEAWAYS ON STRESS

- Chronic stress triggers your immune system. Stress releases inflammatory substances that travel through your body and attack body tissues. Stress causes disease.
- Stress is a cause of leaky gut
- Stress can bring on a flare
- Breathing exercises are critical to releasing stress. They only take a few minutes and should be done several times a day.
- Pause every morning to practice gratefulness.
- Laugh often.
- Learn to say no to others and learn to say yes to you.
- Relax and believe that everything is occurring as it should. Even negative events in our lives open doors to a positive new tomorrow.
- Rumi – "Live life as if everything is rigged in your favor."

Stress, sigh. I have an interesting relationship with stress. Years ago, friends would try and talk to me about the stress I was under and I would laugh. Stress to me was a critical component keeping me on track to accomplish what I wanted to achieve in life.

This was long before I depleted my cortisol to the point that I was almost diseased.

I didn't understand that stress accumulates – and it gathers strength over the years.

I wasn't completely wrong; stress can help you perform under pressure. That is its role. It is there to keep you safe when you are in danger. *Fight or Flight*, adrenaline, and cortisol put the body into action mode. These hormones increase our stamina, increase our reaction time, and enhance our focus. They create energy to meet challenges.

But they are there to work in crisis, not to work in our daily life. We are not being chased by tigers anymore.

When stress is part of our daily life, our body gets out of whack. When it gets out of control, it causes damage, and that damage leads to physical problems.

We put ourselves up against too many deadlines, frustrations, and demands, and no longer realize that we are under a toxic load of stress.[364] [365]

- Chronic stress can shut down our immune system.
- It increases chronic diseases.[366]
- It upsets our digestive system.
- It raises our blood pressure.
- It increases our chances of a heart attack and stroke.
- It fuels cancer in animal studies.
- It causes depression.
- It can shrink our brain.
- It interrupts our sleep.
- It causes us to gain weight.
- It creates an environment for *ANTs*[367] (crazy anxious, negative thoughts, that we use to beat ourselves up with.)
- It breaks down our immune system, and we get colds and the flu more often.
- It prematurely ages kids.[368]
- It can affect your offspring's' genes.
- Stress causes headaches.
- It causes irritability.
- It causes bazaar dreams.[369]
- It can cause jaw pain.
- It can cause hair loss.[370]

Chronic stress is not pretty, and it's not fun to be around.

The adrenals are the body's shock absorbers. Adrenaline, DHEA, and Cortisol control blood sugar, blood pressure, and many other functions of the body. When they get out of whack, they can't fulfill their mission. Stress depletes your cortisol and your DHEA.

But worst of all, stress triggers your immune system. Stress releases inflammatory substances that travel through your body and attack body tissues. Over time, it exasperates leaky gut. And left unbridled, stress causes disease.

Belly fat signals adrenal fatigue; the body stores fat preparing for an impending disaster. The body *wants* to make sure it is prepared. There are tons of cortisol receptors in our belly fat.

To this day, after working on lowering my stress now for five years, if I get super stressed, it can cause a "flare." A flare is where my body attacks me again; I can gain 5 pounds overnight, all of my muscle and joint aches return; the fire gets fueled for my autoimmune issues.

So, if you are struggling with inflammation, you absolutely must do something about your stress. The stress can kill you.

A ground breaking new book *The Telomere Effect: A Revolutionary Approach to Living Younger, Healthier, Longer* by Elizabeth Blackburn, PhD and Elissa Epel, PhD, **Grand Central Publishing** (January 3, 2017) is a book co-authored by the Nobel Prize winner who discovered telomerase and telomeres' role in the aging process; and the health psychologist who has done original research into how specific lifestyle and psychological habits can protect telomeres, slowing disease and improving life.

In this book, they state:

"Your telomeres don't sweat the small stuff. Toxic stress, on the other hand, is something to watch for. Toxic stress is severe stress that lasts for years. Toxic stress can dampen down telomerase and shorten telomeres. Short telomeres create sluggish immune function and make you vulnerable even to catching the common cold. Short telomeres promote inflammation (particularly in the CD8 T-cells), and the slow rise of inflammation leads to degeneration of our tissues and diseases of aging. We cannot rid ourselves of stress, but approaching stressful events with a challenge mentality can help promote protective stress resilience in body and mind."

Finding ways to reframe stress in our lives is crucial to reversing inflammation and also to squelching the degeneration of our tissues and the diseases of aging. Powerful stuff.

I think a little explanation of my history might be helpful to you.

My first Doctor of Chiropractic discovered that my cortisol was very low. This was caused by years of chronic stress.

We already knew that I had undefined autoimmune disease, which my conventional doctor did not acknowledge. I had all of the markers, but my conventional doctor didn't run the test, or maybe know what test to run.

My first Doctor of Chiropractic ran the test, but my conventional doctor didn't acknowledge the results. When I showed my conventional doctor my test for cortisol, since it was very low, but not in a diseased state, she did not see it as an issue. To humor me, she sent me to the Endocrinology Department. We ran a series of tests and yes, the result was cortisol was low, but I wasn't in a diseased state, so nothing to do. I had onset Adrenal Fatigue, but they did not respond.

When I went to my new Functional MD, she immediately saw it as an issue. She started me on **Metagenics "Adreset"** which is an herbal supplement for stress related fatigue. Then we did a test on my DHEA levels, which were completely depleted. Cortisol is made from DHEA, but I didn't have sufficient DHEA to make cortisol. I was given a DHEA spray to use twice a day in my mouth. When we tested two months later, my DHEA had started to replenish, and my cortisol level began to creep back up. I had more energy; I felt better.

Listen to your body. You know when there is a problem so don't take no for an answer. If need be, get a second opinion.

So, what can you do to correct your stress level long term?

First of all, eating clean, with lots of yummy veggies of all colors of the rainbow is core to having good hormones. That is always the first place to start.

Next, relax and believe that everything is occurring as it should; even negative events in our lives open doors to a positive new tomorrow.

"Live life as if everything is rigged in your favor."

RUMI

Then, I do two things when I first get up in the morning.

The first thing I do every morning is a breathing exercise from **Dr. Andrew Weil's** website.

The 4-7-8 (or Relaxing Breath) Exercise[371]

"This breathing exercise is utterly simple, takes almost no time, requires no equipment and can be done anywhere. Although you can do the exercise in any position, sit with your back straight while learning the exercise. Place the tip of your tongue against the ridge of tissue just behind your upper front teeth, and keep it there through the entire exercise. You will be exhaling through your mouth around your tongue; try pursing your lips slightly if this seems awkward.

- "Exhale completely through your mouth, making a whoosh sound.
- "Close your mouth and inhale quietly through your nose to a mental count of **four**. Make sure you are breathing from your belly, and not your chest.
- "Hold your breath for a count of **seven**.
- "Exhale completely through your mouth, making a whoosh sound to a count of **eight**.
- "This is one breath. Now inhale again and repeat the cycle three more times for a total of four breaths."

Breathe in quietly through your nose, breath from your belly, not from your chest, and breathe out audibly through your mouth. The speed of the exercise is not important but the ratio is important. Over time you can slow it down.

If I find myself in a stressful situation, then I also do this exercise. When I am in heavy traffic, I relax using this breathing technique, even if I am going to be late for an appointment. (I travel an hour each way to my doctor's office. Last week there was an accident. So, I started to fret that I was going to be late. I started doing this breathing exercise in the car. When I finally arrived, I did it again in the waiting room. When the nurse took my blood pressure, my pulse was very calm and slow. This started a conversation with my doctor who generally does not observe this in her patients. The breathing exercise works.)

I also do this breathing exercise if I can't fall asleep at night. It immediately relaxes me.

The second thing I do every morning is I make a list of 10-12 things I am grateful for, at that moment in time. It focuses my brain on the many wonderful things I have in my life and helps me stay away from negativity.

I have also discovered a Tao Korean Belly Button Wand. The theory is that since our belly button is our original source of life, if we massage that area with the belly button wand, using gentle vibrations, and if we direct the wand in the direction of our different organs, we can exercise the organ and start to heal the body. The technique has been tested with brain scans, and the mind becomes very calm after only 10 minutes of doing the belly button exercise. It is important to remember to breathe in slowly through your nose, and breathe out slowly through your mouth while you are doing the exercise. It's very relaxing. This does the following:[372]

1. "Promoted blood circulation
2. "Warms the abdomen, increasing body temperature
3. "Improves digestive and excretory functions
4. "Relaxes the body and mind
5. "Increases immunity and detoxification
6. "Boosts physical vitality
7. "Clears the head and improves concentration
8. "Relieves pain and tension in joints
9. "Expands physical and mental well-being
10. "Makes the skin lustrous and smooth
11. "Creates feelings of centeredness."

There are many ways to relax throughout the day. These are some of my favorites. You can pick and choose on a daily basis. Remember, you MUST do something, every day, to release your stress.

- Increase my magnesium to reduce stress, when necessary
- I take a hot Epsom salt bath with lavender oil at the end of almost every day. They aren't long baths, but long enough to wash the troubles of the day away. I add a little argon oil to soften my skin.
- I get up and stretch for 2-3 minutes every 2 hours or so, to stay limber and relieve stress points
- I relax for 10 minutes mid-day with my two cats. They are always thrilled with the attention and my love for them calms and relaxes me.

- I take a chamomile tea break every afternoon. Chamomile relaxes the body and soothes the soul
- I put essential oils in my diffuser in my living room. The aroma brings me pleasure.
- I buy flowers and put them on my dining room table. They make me happy.
- I try to bring laughter, humor and joy into my life every day.
- I get a long hug every morning and every evening from my honey. The hug soothes my soul.
- I try and do a random act of kindness whenever the opportunity arises.
- Nod in with a friend. I have friends now all over the country and I try to nod in at least every two weeks. A heart to heart with a girlfriend is worth its weight in gold.
- I get 7 hours of sleep at night, which has done wonders for my stress level.
- I get a massage every two weeks, a treat from my adorable husband. We get doubles massages to keep us both stress-free.
- The two of us take Tao Yoga 3 times a week. **(Body and Brain)** It's a lovely class with Thai Chi movement, resistance, stretching, and we do move enough for me to break out in a sweat.
- The other days of the week, I jump on my rebounder, which I call my mini trampoline. I record the top 20 country western hits of the week on Sunday and then jump to that recording for 30 minutes. It cleanses the sludge out of my lymph system and gets my heart beat going.
- Meditation, I try and do it for 15 minutes a couple of times a week. I just heard a lecture in school that it is important to Meditate every day for 10 minutes, and that it will reduce stress and lower my blood pressure. I will work on this.
- Although I am diabetic, I have a square of 70% dark chocolate every day. It's my sweet treat.
- Journal, we will discuss this further in Chapter 24 on *ANTs*.
- Watch TV with your honey, relax.
- Eat dinner (usually home cooked) with your honey and share the highlights of your day.

Other things that might be right for you

- Take a long walk in nature several times a week.
- Light candles.
- Play classical music.
- Go to the gym.
- Put on music and dance around your living room for 15 minutes.
- Squeeze a stress ball.
- Read – I love to read, but am very busy at the moment writing this book. I will add it back into my routine when this book is finished.
- If you live away from your family, call them at least once a week and tell them you love them.
- Acknowledge and expose yourself to your fears; then face them down. They won't stress you out anymore.

A couple more thoughts:

- Laugh often. One moment of anger weakens the immune system for 5 hours. One moment of laughter boosts the immune system for 24 hours[373]. Laughter is an amazing stress buster.
- Accept what you cannot change.
- Leave time for the unexpected. If I get somewhere early, I have a complete entertainment system on my phone, and can grab a few moments to read or catch up with emails.
- Don't say yes to everything and everyone. This is part of loving yourself and self-care. You are just as important as anyone else, and your needs always should come first.
- Choose your relationships carefully. My next chapter is on toxic relationships (Part 5, Chapter 23).

Stop overcommitting yourself. It's ok to take care of you, and to say NO!

"You have to learn to say no without feeling guilty. Setting boundaries is healthy. You need to learn to respect and take care of yourself."

UNKNOWN AWESOMEQUOTES4U.COM

Finally, I want you to be kind to you. Practice kind thoughts about yourself. I had a severe case of "not enough". I wasn't good enough to find the right guy. I wasn't good enough to land the big customer; I was too fat; I was too something else. It haunted me daily. Those are *ANTs* (Part 5, Chapter 24), and they do you no good, but they do increase your stress level which does your body harm.

How should you eat to reduce stress? Heal your gut strategies also work here.

1. I eat very clean (lots of organic vegetables, only grass fed meat, wild seafood, (avoids the stress hormone from the factory farmed animals) no junk food, no processed food, and no fast food.) I find cooking at home to be very relaxing and have become quite the short order cook.

2. Cut out the coffee and replace it with hot lemon water in the morning. I find it just as satisfying, and it's important for your adrenals that you don't get extra stimulation.

3. Reduce sugar. Your body can't utilize it, and it gets all whacked out from the sugar. It's important to remove the sugar from your diet to heal your gut.

4. Eat naturally occurring fats: ghee, and coconut, avocado, and olive oils are all good choices.

5. Eat more clean protein, either grass-fed (grass-finished) meat or if vegan, organic soy, and beans.

"Investing in yourself is the best investment you will ever make. It will not only improve your life; it will improve the lives of all of those around you."

ROBIN S. SHARMA

Good health is about the joy of finding the life that you have always wanted but didn't know how to get. Reducing stress is a giant step in the right direction. If you don't reduce your chronic stress it will shorten your life.

UNLESS YOU ARE BEING CHASED BY A TIGER, OR IT'S EQUIVILENT, STRESS SERVES YOU NO PURPOSE. GET RID OF IT NOW, TODAY. Let it go – do the exercises noted above.

Chapter 23

Toxic Relationships

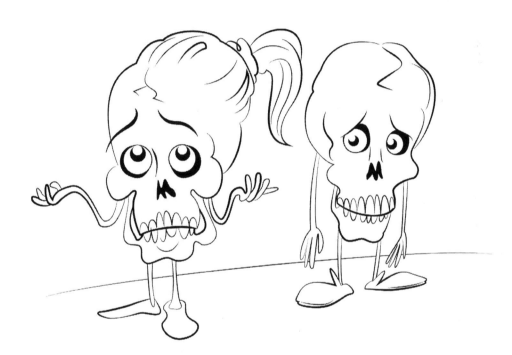

Dousing the flame of inflammation:

THE BIG TAKEAWAYS ON TOXIC RELATIONSHIPS

- Staying in a toxic relationship makes the stress continual, whether it's a toxic love relationship, a toxic friendship or a toxic parent.
- Try to talk to this loved one to improve the relationship and put a plan together. If it can't happen, either walk away (friendship or love relationship) or set boundaries (parent.). It's literally killing you.
- When you are suffering from inflammation, you need to turn your loving attention to yourself, to get well.
- Reach out to close friends for loving support if you have ended a toxic love relationship. You need unconditional love right now to improve your health.
- Walk away with no regrets.
- Make a list of all of the amazing qualities you have and read them every day. Have close friends help you.

"You don't ever have to feel guilty about removing toxic people from your life. It doesn't matter whether someone is a relative, romantic interest, employer, childhood friend, or a new acquaintance – you don't have to make room for people who cause you pain or make you feel small. It's one thing if a person owns up to their behavior and makes an effort to change, but if a person disregards your feelings, ignores your boundaries, and 'continues' to treat you in a harmful way, they need to go."

DANIELL KOEPKE

Toxic relationships can make you ill, whether it's a toxic love relationship, a toxic friendship, a toxic employer, or a toxic relative.

Significant Other Relationships

I was in a relationship for nine years that started out healthy. He helped me start my jewelry business; he wrote my operating system, and he paid for all of my food and all of my entertainment for years while I was getting started. I am very grateful to him, and I loved him very much. In the beginning, and then in many of the years that followed, he was extraordinarily good to me.

He loved to go out to expensive restau*rants*. But after being together for eight years, when I got diabetes and wanted to stop eating out every night for heavy calorie laden food, my significant other announced that he didn't like it that I was diabetic.

What was I supposed to do with that?

He didn't want me to cook home cooked meals. He didn't want me to dictate what he was going to eat each night.

He was upset that I had gained weight, a lot of weight, and he blamed me for the weight he had gained. (We had eaten our way through Pasadena, and he had gained weight too.)

Furthermore, after time, this guy didn't appreciate me for who I was, he only saw me for who I was not.

He had recently lost a lot of money in the stock market and had become sullen and difficult to be around. He started dating other women, unbeknownst to me.

These were all just symptoms of the underlying toxicity that was growing.

I would have never left him when he was down, but he did me a big favor when he left me.

There is no doubt that he broke my heart, but as I came out the other side of my pain, I realized I could start to deal with the pain my body was experiencing; that the inflammation in my body had begun. I could start to eat the way I was supposed to for my diabetes and sugar control; I could start to take care of me. In the end, I understand that he did me a big favor, and the break-up set me on the road to health.

In the first eight months, I lost 40 pounds.

I took a class on how to date from **Allison Armstrong** (an amazing guru with very sensible advice on dating) and nine months later I met an amazing guy by doing a profile on the dating service **Our Time.com**. Using what I learned from Allison's seminars, I wrote that I was looking for a guy that would intellectually stimulate me, (John is a statistician), that was kind and had high ethics, and he needed to be open to eating home cooked food that was organic and healthy. He needed to want to live an entirely healthy lifestyle.

The guy that answered lived 10 minutes away from me and two years ago, I married him.

John just *wants* me to be happy. He was married for 42 years to a therapist, and she died from cancer after being ill for five years. He loved her very much. He was ready for a new life experience, and lucky me, he chose to find that experience with me.

He is a true partner and supports me in all that I do. He is easy going, and he sees me for who I am, and doesn't criticize me for who I am not.

He completely supports me in my quest for health, and he has lost 70 pounds in the time we have been together. He considers himself my first Health Coaching success.

I have tons of sensitivities, and each time my doctor and I uncovered more, and I lost new foods to eat, John's response was "It's ok, honey, we can just invent a new way to cook." God love him.

I am telling you my story because if you are in a toxic love relationship, sit down and talk it out in an attempt to change course and make it better. It that is impossible, then get out. Get out now, and take care of yourself. There is someone wonderful at the other end of the dark cloud. And if you don't get out, you will not be able to give the attention to yourself that you need to start to heal, which is the most important thing that you can do for yourself.

So, let's define what a toxic relationship is. (They don't necessarily have to be love interests, they could be toxic friends, or even a toxic parent or relative, or even a toxic employer. But they need to be purged, none the less)

Any of these issues are toxic, and you need to think about the relationship in those terms.

Signs of toxic people:

- They are never wrong.
- They love the drama, or are completely shut down and show no drama at all.
- They are constantly critical.
- They like to talk and interrupt.
- They lack compassion.
- They love to gossip and talk badly about others.
- They are into negativity.
- They isolate you from others.

Signs of toxic behavior:[375]

- They are passive-aggressive.
- They are displaying jealousy and the blame-game.
- They are showing criticism and contempt.
- They are exuding tons of negative energy.
- You can't seem to do anything right.
- They are avoiding you.
- Neither of you is happy anymore, but they are making no effort to improve things.

In an article in WikiHow called **How to Recognize a Toxic Friend**, [376] they point out the following:

"If you think you are in a toxic friendship, consider your feelings about your friend and the time spent together, and ask yourself these questions:

- "Is this something that your friend has just started to do, or has it been going on for a long time?
- "Do you feel unhappy after spending time with this friend? Does spending time with your friend make you feel defensive or upset?
- "Do you spend time justifying your own behavior around your friend instead of it feeling 'natural' to be together?
- "Are you happy with this friend?
- "Do you feel belittled, attacked or used?

- "Does the friendship feel unbalanced and like plain hard work?
- "Do you feel at fault for things that happen to your friend?
- "Has your friend betrayed your confidences?
- "Does it feel like competition rather than a balanced and caring friendship?"

If you are in a toxic relationship, you must sit down and talk to your friend, lover or parent. Set boundaries, and see if you can save the relationship. If not, you need to walk away. You must reduce your stress, and be with people you are grateful to have in your life. If you are in a toxic relationship with a parent or relative, setting boundaries is crucial. Talk to them about the relationship and what you need. If it is a toxic employer, ask for a transfer or find a new position with a healthier environment.

These are words of wisdom from Kris Carr of **Sexy, Crazy, Cancer**.[377]

From her blog on her website: ***"How to Identify & Release Toxic Relationships"***

"No matter who you are in a toxic relationship with these are questions to ponder: (Most likely you won't feel all of them)

- "Is the pain too great to stay the same?
- "Do I constantly picture an alternate reality?
- "Do I need a translator to be heard?
- "Is it impossible to make boundaries?
- "Am I the only one that is willing to meet in the middle?
- "Is getting an apology (when it's truly deserved) like pulling teeth?
- "Does this relationship take more energy than it gives?
- "Is blaming and complaining getting really old?
- "Am I completely fatigued when I'm with the person and energetic when they're gone?

"If it's a romantic relationship –

- "Are the sparks between the two of you dead – end of story?
- "Do I smile when I want to yell, and then yell at the wrong people?
- "Is the only thing holding me back my fear of newness?
- "Am I afraid of what people will think of me if this relationship fails?
- "Does this person make me feel like I'm lost without them?

- "Do I find myself missing the old me?
- "Am I lonely even when I am with him (or her)?"

There are two significant problems with staying in any toxic relationship, toxic love, toxic friendship or toxic parent. The stress is killing you, and the relationship is zapping all of the energy out of you, energy that needs to be directed to helping you get well.

If you decide to end a toxic love relationship, reach out for support. You will need unconditional love while you go through the heartbreak. No matter how difficult the relationship has become, if you love him (or her), it will be very painful to pull away.

When you end any toxic relationship, walk away gracefully with no regrets. No accusations. No, if only you had done this. No manipulation, no finger pointing. (And if leaving toxic employment, no bridge burning.)

Once free, write down all the things that you are truly grateful for from being in that relationship and set those memories free. Holding onto your grudges will do you no good and does them no harm. Let it go and start to heal. Life has many wonderful adventures waiting for you, but you have to be free and clear to pull them in.

Make sure you take the time to write down all of the things that are wonderful about you. Ask your dearest friends to help you make a list. What happened isn't your fault, it's not anyone's fault. It's just time to move on.

I learned a long time ago; sometimes there is an Angel's hand on my back leading me away from one place to another, where I am supposed to be, where I can find joy and happiness. Getting out of any toxic relationship is an angel's hand on your back moving you to a better place where you can find health and happiness.

Chapter 24

"ANTs"

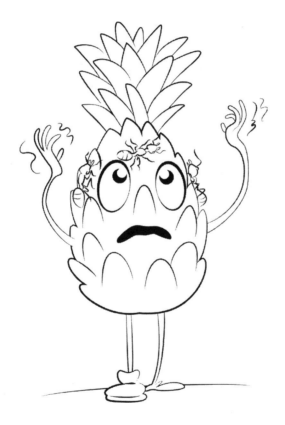

(Annoying little thoughts in your mind.) *ANTs**[379] is a term coined by Dr. Daniel G. Amen for "**Anxious Negative Thoughts.**"

Dousing the flame of inflammation:

THE BIG TAKEAWAYS ON *ANTs*

- Don't believe everything you think. Most of your negative thoughts are not true.
- Write your negative thoughts down, investigate whether or not they are true, and then talk back.
- Dr. Amen states that every thought produces a chemical. If you focus on negative thoughts, not only will it ruin your day, and impact your relationships, long term it can even ruin your memory.[380]
- Post my wisdom phrases somewhere you can readily read them, on your computer, on the wall of your office, somewhere within eyesight. Read them when the *ants* start to multiply.
- Practice Morning pages or
- Practice the "thank your body meditation" when you first wake up

ANTs – What are they and how do you kill them off?

I love the term. I hate it when real *ants* invade my kitchen. Toxic thoughts are just like that.

All of a sudden, you don't know where the crack is that is letting them in, but they seem to be everywhere. These "Automatic Negative Thoughts," in my case, are also known as worry, lots and lots of worry, and negative thoughts about me, with a big dose of fear, and insecurity. All these thoughts are buried under the surface. A lot of if only, then I could … you know, "Coulda, wouldas." I had a healthy dose of "*ANTs**" when I started my get-well journey, and I am now, relatively, ANT Free.

As a start, don't listen to everything your mind tells you. It is not the truth. It's just some idle chatter to keep you in your "already always."[381] It tears you down so that you stay in your old known truth, even if it is false, which has become your comfort zone. As you open up your possibilities, these *ANTs* no longer serve you. In fact, they never did.

This is how Dr. Amen describes *ANTs* in an article in April Showers, August 29, 2014, **9 Types of Automatic Negative Thoughts**:

"*ANTs** fall into these categories:[382]

"All or nothing – These are the *ANTs* that infest your brain when you think everything is all good or all bad. It is the same as black or white thinking. If you stick to your exercise plan for a month, you think you are the most disciplined person on the planet. If you miss a day at the gym, you think you have no discipline and give up and go back to being a coach potato. A better approach is to acknowledge that you didn't do your daily workout and then get back on track the following day. One slip up doesn't mean you should give up entirely.

1. "Always thinking – This is when you think in words that over generalize, such as always, never, every time or everyone. Consider some of the thoughts such as 'I will never lose weight,' 'I have always had a sweet tooth – I will never be able to stop eating chocolate,' This kind of thinking makes you feel like you are doomed to fail at eating right and staying healthy. It is as if you have no control over your actions or behaviors.

2. "Focusing on the negative – This ANT makes you see only the negative aspects of situations even when there are plenty of positives. 'I know I lost 10 pounds, but I wanted to lose 15, so I'm a failure' is an example of this type of thinking. Focusing on the negative makes you more inclined to give up on your efforts. Putting a positive spin on this same thought, – "wow!" I lost 10 pounds. I'm on my way to my goal of 15 pounds' – encourages you to keep up the good work and makes you feel pretty good about yourself.

3. "Thinking with your feelings – 'I feel like my skin is never going to clear up.' Thoughts like this occur when you have a feeling about something and you assume it is correct, so you never question it. Feelings can lie too. Look for evidence. In this example, schedule an appointment with a dermatologist to find out if there's anything you can do to improve your skin.

4. "Guilt beating – Thinking in words like 'should,' 'must', 'ought to,' and 'have to' are typical with this type of ANT, which involves using excessive guilt to control behavior. When we feel pushed to do things, our natural tendency is to push back. That doesn't mean that guilt is all bad. There are certainly things in life that we should and shouldn't do if we want to have the best body possible: 'I want to eat the chips and guacamole at the party, but

I should have the raw carrots instead' or 'I feel like staying in bed, but I should do my workout.' Don't mistake these for guilt beating *ANTs*.

5. "Labeling – When you call yourself or someone else names or use negative terms to describe them, you have a labeling ANT in your brain. A lot of us do this on a regular basis. You may have said one of the following at some point in your life; 'I'm a loser'; 'I'm a failure'; or 'I'm lazy.' The problem with calling yourself names is that it takes away your actions and behaviors. If you are a loser, a failure, or lazy, then why bother trying to change your behavior? It is as if you have given up before you have even tried. This defeatist attitude can be ruinous for your body."

"Beware of the red *ANTs**:"

These last three *ANTs** are the worst of the bunch. Dr. Amen calls them the red *ANTs* because they can really sting.

1. "Fortune telling – Predicting the worst even though you don't know what will happen is the hallmark of the fortune telling ANT*. Examples include: 'I just had a biopsy I am sure it is cancer.' Nobody is safe from fortune telling *ANTs**.

2. "Mind reading – When you think that you know what somebody else is thinking even though they have not told you, and you have not asked them, it is called mind-reading. Listen carefully to the other person before trying to predict what they have to say.

3. "Blame – Of all the *ANTs**, this one is the worst. Blaming others for your problems and taking no responsibility for your own successes and failures is toxic thinking. For example: 'It is your fault I'm out of shape because you will not go with me to exercise.' Whenever you begin a sentence with 'it is your fault ...' it ruins your life. These *ANTs* make you a victim. When you are a victim, you are powerless to change your behavior. Quit blaming others and take responsibility for your actions."

A few of my favorite phrases of wisdom about *ANTs** and worry:

"You don't need to change your negative thoughts; you just need to change how you engage with then. Observe them, and then let them naturally pass like clouds in the sky. They will pass, they always do."

LORI DESCHANE

"Don't believe everything you think; thoughts are just that, thoughts."

ALLAN LOKOS

"You don't have to control your thoughts. You just have to stop letting them control you."

DAN MILLMAN

"Worry does not take away tomorrow's troubles. It takes away today's peace."

UNKNOWN

"Worry is like walking around with an umbrella waiting for it to rain."

UNKNOWN

"No amount of anxiety makes any difference to anything that is going to happen."

ALAN WATTS

"Worry is a down payment on a problem you many never have."

JOYCE MEYER

However, it ends up; I inherited some of my worry. I know that my Mother had *ANTs*, and I inherited the same chemical imbalance that she had to get my own invasion.

To begin with, under the guidance of my functional MD, I take a new supplement, and it quieted the beast. It is called **Trancor**, for balance and relaxation by **Metagenics**.

That was a good start. But I have also developed some techniques that have kept *ANTs* at bay.

Dr. Amen makes the following suggestions:[383]

"When you are sad, mad, and nervous or out of control,[384] or thinking unkind thoughts about yourself:

1. "Write it down. When those automatic negative thoughts start tumbling around in your mind, write them down to clearly identify them.

2. "Investigate. Ask yourself, are these thoughts even true? Uninvestigated thoughts can lead us to act in harmful ways.

3. "Talk back. If you discover that these negative thoughts are false, talk back to them! Tell these thoughts you know they aren't true!"

He also recommends a supplement that he developed to calm the *ANTs** – **Gaba Calming Support**.

I took a course called **Investment in Excellence**[385] years ago. They recommended when you thought nasty things about yourself, you immediately reply to yourself, "Why would you say that about yourself, Cheryl. You know that is not true." I began to turn my *ANTs** around by using that method.

Dr. Amen continues that every thought produces a chemical. If you focus on negative thoughts, not only will it ruin your day, and impact your relationships, long term it can even ruin your memory. Wow! Where is the ant spray?

Next thing I do that has been useful:

I try and do **Morning Pages**[386] three mornings a week for ½ an hour. It's my secret treat. I get up early, so before I check my email or Facebook, I open up my journal and free write. I don't control my thoughts; I write whatever comes off my pen. This is a technique developed by Julia Cameron to cultivate creativity and personal growth. For me, it is a secret pleasure.

Sometimes I write coherently – things I need to accomplish in the day, things I am grateful for, affirmations I want to repeat for my future.

Sometimes my thoughts are dark thoughts, but by writing them down, I can sweep them away for the rest of the day.

Julia recommends that you write down what you remember of your dreams. I rarely remember my dreams, so I still need to develop that muscle.

Sometimes my thoughts are creative, and I find a new direction for a task that I am undertaking.

Often, I concentrate on what deserves gratitude. It starts my day off on a positive foot.

The idea is that you do this before you are fully awake and before your ego becomes fully present. The idea is to tap into your subconscious mind. It has helped me kill off the *ANTs*. If they need to appear, they appear here, and I sweep them away. This journal is for you. No one else will ever read it, so write away in the privacy of your own mind and journal.

Another exercise I have learned, when I wake up in the morning, before I get up, (In lieu of Morning Papers) I say good morning to each part of my body. It's a lovely exercise that I learned on a Tao retreat in Sedona called Sedona Mago Retreat. (Which I strongly recommend to relax and feed your soul in a perfect spot, with amazing energy from the vortex's, with beautiful pescatarian food and wise sages.)[387]

- Sit up in bed and start with your feet and say Good Morning feet. How are you today? "Thank you so much for being my feet and for supporting me all of my life." While you are saying that, massage your feet for several seconds and then tap on them hard to wake them up and get the blood circulating.
- Move up to your calves and go through the same routine, "Good morning calves how are you today? Thank you so much for being my calves and for supporting me all of my life."
- Next your thighs, same routine.
- Then massage your belly button. Spend extra time here, being grateful for your belly button, since it was your beginning source of life. Say good morning belly button, thank it for being your original source of life and give your belly button extra love and massage and then tap to wake it up and get the blood circulating.
- Now go to your solar plexus, then up to your heart, then your hands, your arms, your neck, your face, your top of your head. Thank each part of you, and rub and massage it with love, and then tap it, waking it up and giving it loving energy.

This exercise allows me to start my day in peace and joy.

At first, this felt silly, but it brings me a source of contentment to start my day. And best of all, it tames the *ANTs* and sets my mind free.

One last thought about *ANTs*:*

If your inner critic is working overtime in your brain, invite your inner champion to take its place.[388]

Write down what your inner champion is saying to stifle the inner critic until it can't get air. Let your inner champion "crowd" out your inner critic. Kill off those inner critic thoughts like weeds. You deserve thoughts that admire and defend you.

Plant your champion thoughts and let them grow.

"It takes but one positive thought when given a chance to survive and thrive, to overpower an entire army of negative thoughts."

ROBERT H. SCHULLER (FROM DEANNA MINICH.COM[389])

Chapter 25

Toxic lack of sleep and what to do about it

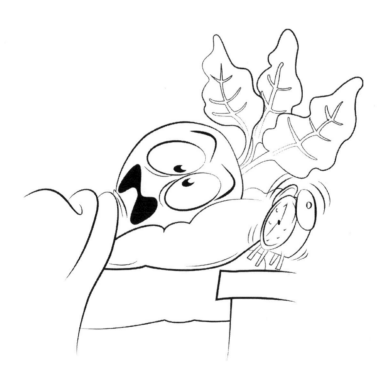

301

Dousing the flame of inflammation:

THE BIG TAKEAWAYS ON SLEEP

- 7-8 hours of sleep a night is critical especially if you have inflammation
- Sleep is the #1 health problem in the United States, affecting 100 million people.[391]
- The brain, according to Dr. Rubin Naiman PHD, (Sleep expert) is the second gut.
- Sleeping recharges your immune system.
- Important body functions take place while you are asleep.
- There are 32 suggestions in this chapter from leading experts to help you fall asleep.
- Eating clean, with lots of yummy vegetables in every color of the rainbow, is just as important to sleep as it is to everything else happening in your body. It also creates a happy environment for a calm digestive system which encourages sleep. It is crucial to your life.

"Get at least eight hours of beauty sleep a night; nine if you're ugly"

BETTY WHITE TO DAVID LETTERMAN (I HAD TO INCLUDE THIS, I THINK IT'S A RIOT)

This is an interesting chapter to write, because usually, I don't have a problem sleeping. My husband told me, he had to get used to the fact that I come to bed, and he is mid-sentence as my head hits the pillow, and I am out. (We are newlyweds.)

As I grow older, though, I do have a problem getting to sleep on occasion, so at the end of this article, I will discuss what I do about it.

Most of my friends, however, have a terrible time with sleep. I used to think I should develop a phone with lights so that if you were awake in the middle of the night, you would know who else in your life was awake so that you could call and chat. It would have been a bit hit with my friends.

It makes sense to me to learn that sleep is the #1 health problem in America, affecting 100 million people.[392]

So, let's talk about sleep, why it is so important, what causes the inability to fall asleep right away, and then what to do about it.

First of all, the standard is 7-8 hours of sleep a night; less than 7 hours is where the trouble begins.

Sleep is critical if you are having an issue with inflammation. More than anyone else, getting 7-8 hours of sleep is important to douse the fire.

In an article called ***What Happens When You Sleep***.[393] From About.com

- "Sleep is when you do repair work in your body, in your heart and your cardiovascular system.
- "Growth, sex, and fertility hormones are released during the sleep cycle.
- "Other sleep cycle hormones help regulate your appetite.
- "Your body temperature falls when sleeping.
- "The digestive system and metabolic rate slow down during sleep."

An article in Science Daily Loss Of Sleep, *Even For A Single Night, Increases Inflammation In The Body* 9/4/2008 states:

"Loss of sleep, even for a few short hours during the night, can prompt one's immune system to turn against healthy tissue and organs. Losing sleep for even part of one night can trigger the key cellular pathway that produces tissue-damaging inflammation according to new research. The findings suggest a good night's sleep can ease the risk of both heart disease and autoimmune disorders such as rheumatoid arthritis."[394]

According to the NIH (National Institute of Health) in an article called *Why Is Sleep Important?* It states:

"The damage from sleep deficiency can occur in an instant (such as a car crash), or it can harm you over time. For example, ongoing sleep deficiency can raise your risk for some chronic health problems. It also can affect how well you think, react, work, learn, and get along with others."[395]

A good night sleep

- Improves your learning.
- Helps you stay creative.
- Helps you pay attention and make decisions.
- Controls your hunger hormones, to balance leptin and ghrelin.
- Supports healthy growth in children.
- Allows your body to repair cells.
- Your blood pressure drops while you sleep.
- Increases blood supply to your muscles, especially important if you have been injured.[396]
- Recharges your immune system and quells inflammation.
- Reboots your brain

You have heard that your gut is your second brain. Did you know that your brain is your second gut? "Imagine the brain as a second gut," says Rubin Naiman, Ph.D., a clinical psychologist specializing in integrative sleep and dream medicine at the University of Arizona. "At night, the brain metaphorically swallows, digests and sifts through information, and, just like the gut, eliminates," he says. In an article called *"9 Things You Probably Didn't Know About Dreaming"* in **The Huffington Post** 2/24/2014.

If you're sleep deficient, (less than 7 hours) you may have trouble –

- Making decisions.
- Solving problems.
- Controlling your emotions and behavior.
- Coping with change.

In addition, a lack of sleep:

- Is linked to depression, suicide, and risk-taking behavior.[397]
- Causes inflammation and can cause an autoimmune flare.[398]
- Causes a lower blood flow to the brain.[399]
- Creates mood swings; you become angry and impulsive.[400]
- Increases your chances of obesity.[401]

- Creates moments of micro sleep, and you may not even be aware of it. Micro sleep is where you nod off briefly, and miss what happened in those moments, at a lecture, watching TV, or at a movie.[402] *(I suffer from micro sleep and didn't even realize it until researching for this book. Recognizing the problem is the first step in fixing it.)*
- Is linked to an increased risk of heart disease, kidney disease, high blood pressure, diabetes, and stroke.[403]
- Increases blood sugar, which increases your risk of diabetes[404]

Things that can interfere with sleep, from Dr. Mark Hyman MD, in his article *8 Ways to Ensure A Better Night's Sleep* in **EcoWatch** 4/16/2016[405]

- "Food sensitivities,
- "Thyroid problems,
- "Menopause,
- "Fibromyalgia,
- "Chronic fatigue syndrome,
- "Heavy metal toxicity,
- "Stress
- "Sleep disorders. Consider getting tested.
    - o "If you suspect deeper issues like sleep apnea, I also recommend **The 8-Hour Sleep Paradox** written by my friend and colleague, Dr. Mark Burhenne. This book dives deep into causes of fatigue and sleep troubles while providing excellent tips and tools for better sleep immediately."

I have put together a variety of sleep suggestions from sleep experts for you to try if sleep is an issue for you. Remember, sleep is an issue if you are not getting at least 7 hours of sleep a night.

Phoenix Helix[406], in an article called ***Can Skipping Sleep Cause an Autoimmune Flare?*** By Eileen (who has autoimmune disease) January 21, 2015 *(I, Cheryl have annotated this quote)*

- "Make the hour before bedtime, quiet time.
- "Avoid strenuous exercise 3 hours before sleep.

- "Eliminate bright artificial light, such as a TV or computer screen. The light signals the brain it's time to wake." (*Cheryl – I use amber sunglasses if I am using these devices the hour before bed.*)
- "Avoid heavy meals 3 hours before bedtime. A light snack is fine. Avoid alcohol before bed.
- "Avoid nicotine, (cigarettes) and caffeine-caffeinated soda, coffee, and tea. The effects of caffeine last as long as 8 hours." (*Cheryl – when I do have coffee, my cut-off time is noon. Otherwise it does keep me awake*)
- "Keep your bedroom quiet, cool and dark." (Cheryl – I turn the heat down to 68 before I go to bed.)
- "Take a hot bath before you go to sleep." (Cheryl – I recommend Epsom salts and lavender. I also add a little argon oil. I have taken baths before bed for the last 30 years, and they probably are a big reason that I sleep so well.)
- "If you have joint pain, consider using extra pillows. Hugging a pillow takes the pressure off your shoulders, and a pillow between your knees takes the pressure off your hips."
- As your Health Muse, I, Cheryl, recommend an essential oil cream made with coconut oil with Frankincense and Mint and a potpourri of other oils rubbed into your joints where you have pain before going to sleep. I have also found topical Magnesium spray to help reduce tension and soreness and keep it next to my bed in case I get a cramp in the middle of the night.

From Dr. Mark Hyman MD, in his article *8 Ways to Ensure A Better Night's Sleep* in **EcoWatch** 4/16/2016

"More things to do to improve your sleep:[407]

- "Get on a regular schedule. Going to sleep and waking at the same time each day creates a rhythm for your body. Only use your bed for sleep or romance.
- "Get natural sunlight. Aim for at least 20 minutes of sunshine every day, preferably in the morning, which triggers your brain to release chemicals that regulate sleep cycles.
- "Use an acupressure mat. It helps to stimulate your parasympathetic nervous system and create deep relaxation. Lay on it for about 30 or more minutes before bed.

- "Get grounded. At times, electromagnetic frequencies can impair sleep. I recommend turning off Wi-Fi and keeping all of your electronic devices away from your bed. Create a common area charging station in your home and encourage all your family members to 'check in' their devices before bed.
- "Clear your mind. Everyone knows how something resonating in your mind can hinder sleep. Turning your mind off can become a challenge. Keep a journal or notebook by your bed and write down your to-do list or ruminations before you go to sleep so you can close your eyes and make it less likely for your mind to spin.
- "Perform light stretching or yoga before bed. This yoga relaxes your mind and body. Research shows daily yoga can improve sleep significantly
- "Use herbal therapies. I recommend 300 to 600 milligrams (mg) of passionflower or 320 to 480 mg of valerian root extract before bed. Other natural sleep supplements include melatonin or magnesium. Potato starch mixed into a glass of water before bedtime can also help. Start slowly with one teaspoon and gradually build up the dose. This feeds good gut bacteria and improves blood sugar control while helping you drift into sleep. You can find sleep and other quality supplements in my store.
- "Use relaxation practices. Guided imagery, meditation or deep breathing calm your mind and help you drift into sleep. Try calming essential oils such as lavender, Roman chamomile or ylang-ylang. Many patients get incredible results with my Ultra Calm CD."

From Daniel Amen, MD (Dr. Amen is a physician, double board certified psychiatrist and ten-time New York Times bestselling author) *Do This, Not That: 10 Tips For A Better Night's Sleep*[408]

- "Drink a mixture of warm unsweetened almond milk, with a teaspoon of vanilla (the real stuff, not the imitation) and a few drops of stevia. This drink may increase serotonin in your brain and help you to sleep."
  (Cheryl's note – I use his Restful Sleep Supplement, and for me, it works like a charm.)
- "If you are a worrier, try Dr. Amen's Gaba Calming Support supplement. It calms the *ANTs*" *(Part 5, Chapter 24.)*

- "Try to avoid taking naps if you aren't sleeping. It's important to get onto a regular sleep cycle. Go to bed at the same time each night, and wake up at the same time each morning. This regularity in sleep habit includes weekends.
- "Never go to bed worried or angry. Send a positive text, an email, or set an intention to deal with the issue tomorrow. Write in a journal and let it go. If you forgive the person, you just might end the conflict.
- "Move the clock so that you can't see it. That way you don't get anxious every time you look at the clock."
  (Cheryl's note – I sometimes get up and move to the couch if I can't get to sleep. I seem to be able to drop right off in a different location.)
- "If little noises are keeping you awake, try sound therapy which can induce a very peaceful mood and lull you to sleep. Consider soothing nature sounds, wind chimes, a fan, or soft music. Studies have shown that slower classical music, or any music that has a slow rhythm of 60 to 80 beats per minute, can help with sleep. If you share the room with someone who snores, try wearing ear plugs.
- "Use your bedroom only for sleep or sexual activity. Sexual activity releases many natural hormones, releases muscle tension and boosts a sense of well-being. Adults with healthy sex lives seem to sleep better.
- "Finish exercising at least 4 hours before bed."

Aviva Romm MD and herbalist suggests[409], in a blog on her website **Sleep Well, Naturally: 7 Steps to Great Zzzz's**

"Do your worrying before bed – 'I have my patients start a pro-sleep journal –

"'Any blank notebook will do. One hour before bed they write out all of their worries and concerns, including their to-do list for the next day. Doing this allows you go to sleep with a clearer head.

"'Oh, and did I say vent in there, too? Never go to sleep angry. Even if you do sleep, you'll have rough dreams.

"'After you've done your writing, read something inspirational for a few minutes. I highly recommend Tara Bennet Goleman's *Mind Whispering* as a start. My patients tell me this whole practice works wonders. (Just don't do it in your bedroom!)'"

These are things that I have done to encourage sleep.

- Banana Tea[410]
- Magnolia bark (you can buy this on Amazon)
- Magnesium
- Amber sunglasses. No blue light after 10pm from computers or TV. Amber Sunglasses will block the blue light
- I read somewhere that the key to a good night sleep is lowering the body's core temperature. I lower the house temperature to 68° as I head for bed.
- Breathing, I do the Andrew Weil breathing exercise in the stress chapter (Part 5, Chapter 22). Works like a charm
- I do a mental exercise using light where I visualize light coming in my top chakra, go back and forth, then I mentally take the light to my third eye, in the middle of my forehead and take the light in and out, and then bring the light to my 5th chakra, the throat chakra, which opens front and back and take the light in and out, down to my heart, take the light in and out, down to my solar plexus, and take the light in and out, down to my 2nd chakra, and take it in and out and then out my root chakra, down to the earth, deep into the earth laying roots as the light travels all the way to the core of the earth. The core of the earth is a bright ball of light. Then I pull the light back up, take it through the root system, and then up through my root chakra, let it pour out my 2nd chakra, my solar plexus, my heart chakra, my throat chakra, my 3rd eye, and then have it cascade out of the top of my head, protecting my entire body as it comes down. By now, usually, I am sound asleep.

Let's hear it for a good night's sleep!

Chapter 26

Movement - Removing the toxic sludge

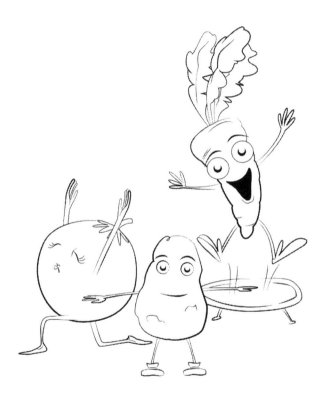

Dousing the flame of inflammation:

THE BIG TAKEAWAYS ON MOVEMENT: REMOVING THE SLUDGE, CREATING FLOW. BALANCING YOUR CHI

- It is important to include gentle exercise into your routine especially if you are suffering from inflammation.
- The form you choose should incorporate resistance (strength), stretching (agility) and aerobic (get the blood flowing and build up muscles like the heart.)
- Movement is essential for detoxification, to move the gook through the lymph system and out of the body.
- Movement releases stress and *ANTs**.
- It encourages many body functions that are inhibited by inflammation: better sleep, a sharper brain, fewer migraines, better skin, and better digestion.
- It creates balance (Chi).
- Movement stirs the soul.
- Movement releases happy hormones (endorphins).

Movement

This has been an issue for me. I have never liked exercise. I wasn't athletic as a child and was always chosen last to be on any sports team. I am not terribly coordinated. It just wasn't my thing. I am a person that lives in my head.

I admit that the times in my life when I exercised regularly, I felt better. But making it a priority to continue, always seemed elusive.

But as I age, and have pain, I understand just how important it is to move.

Movement makes the heart stronger. It moves more oxygen to the muscles and throughout the body. It moves nutrients to the cells. Movement encourages flexibility which decreases pain, and increases agility.

Movement for me has become "self-defense."

In an article called *The Unexpected Side Effects of Exercise*[412] 3/23/2012 in the **Huffington Post**, they state movement improves the following:[413]

- Improved sexual function
- Changes in gene expression
- Better skin
- Healthy eyes
- Better sleep
- A sharper brain
- Fewer Migraines
- Boosted Immunity
- A Sunnier Disposition
- More Birthdays

There are three important elements to movement.

1. Stretching for agility improves muscle elasticity and flexibility. It achieves healthy muscle tone. Stretching improves blood and nutrient flow to muscles; it helps to correct posture. Stretching relieves mental and physical tension.

2. Resistance for strength – it provides bone health and muscle mass. It makes you stronger and fitter. It reduces pain. It releases feel-good hormones (Endorphins). It boosts your energy, improves sleep, it allows your body to burn more calories.

3. Aerobic to make the body stronger and move oxygen. Aerobic exercise burns energy, burns calories, increases stamina, improves the immune system, reduces your health risks for many conditions, heart disease, diabetes, stroke, high blood pressure, and even cancer. It strengthens your heart, keeps your arteries clear, and boosts your mood. It brings you a healthier longer life.

For someone with inflammation or chronic disease, moderate exercise can help reduce stress, and give you a brighter outlook while helping the body to repair.

If you are already exercising regularly, I congratulate you. YEAH! Just make sure it incorporates resistance, stretching and mild aerobic.

If you are not, movement is just as crucial to removing toxins as cleaning up your food and your mind.

You need to find some type of exercise that you can sustain because the health benefits are crucial for a long and healthy life.

I have found two solutions. I call them my "exercise tricks for someone that hates to exercise."

Tao Meditation

This class fulfills my soul on a variety of levels. My husband and I go to classes at **Body and Brain Yoga**. It is pleasant, feel good exercise that involves enough movement to get me to sweat; it incorporates resistance training, and encourages stretching and flexibility. We also work on healing our organs by exercising them through our belly button, with the help of a belly button stick. It is unique, and it works.

I find the classes spiritual; it works with ethereal energy, chakra energy, breathing, stress release, and still gives my body a workout. Both my husband and I enjoy the community of the people in the class. Doing exercise there brings peace and it is a favorite time of my week. It clears the mind of toxins, and "*ANTs**," and encourages energy to move through the body. Movement creates balance (chi), and improves mood. I find the exercise there to be very healing. We are healing my inflammation. We are working on clearing my chakras. The classes are removing the sludge of the soul.

Rebounding

My rebounder is my other secret weapon. I love to rebound. I record the top 20 Country Western hits on Sunday mornings, and then jump to the program all week long. I used to do this with VH1, but they don't have that program on my cable, so I am becoming quite the fan of Country. It's easy to exercise when I am watching videos, and listening to music that I really like.

These are a few of the benefits of rebounding:[414]

- "Increases oxygen to the cells. Where there is oxygen, there can't be disease.
- "Exercises the entire body without additional pressure on the ankles and feet.
- "Rebounding enhances digestion and elimination processes.

- "Rebounding allows for deeper and easier relaxation and sleep.
- "Rebounding results in better mental performance, with keener learning processes.
- "Rebounding curtails fatigue and menstrual discomfort for women.
- "Rebounding minimizes the number of colds, allergies, digestive disturbances, and abdominal problems.
- "Rebounding tends to slow down atrophy in the aging process.
- "Rebounding can actually reverse, prevent or diminish the hardening of the arteries. By conquering this ultimate pathology, you will keep your mind alert, skin smooth, skeleton flexible, libido intact, kidneys functioning, blood circulating, liver detoxifying, enzyme systems alive, hold memory intact, and avoid all systems of the aging process.
- "The up and down motion is very beneficial to the lymph system since the jumping runs vertical to the body.
- "People who rebound find they are able to work longer, sleep better, and feel less tense and nervous. The effect is not just psychological, because the action of bouncing up and down against gravity, without trauma to the musculoskeletal system, is one of the most beneficial aerobic exercises ever developed.
- "It cleans out the sludge from the lymph system. Lymph doesn't have a motor, like the blood has the heart, to move the lymph through its system, so movement is necessary to move it along.
- "Rebounding increases bone mass.
- "Rebounding improves digestion.
- "It is twice as effective as jogging without the impact on ankles and knees.
- "In increases endurance on a cellular level.
- "It helps improve balance by stimulating the vestibule in the middle ear.
- "It circulates oxygen increasing energy.
- "It improves muscle tone.
- "The up and down motion supports the adrenals and thyroid."[415]

And the best answer is that rebounding (which I call my mini trampoline) is FUN! So, I am much more likely to do it.

The last great benefit of movement is that it stirs the soul; it clears the mind, and it makes the body feel great. It releases endorphins. It is well worth the effort, and necessary for a happy, healthy life.

Part 6

Get Involved

Chapter 27

Spread the Word! Organizations to follow and support

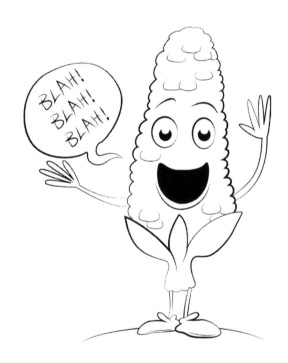

SPREAD THE WORD

It is more important than ever to get involved. The current government is shutting down what little regulation our government had to monitor agriculture, pesticides, pharmaceuticals, big food etc.

The only way we will save ourselves, our children, our planet, is to vote with our dollars. Do not buy the toxic foods outlined in this book, do not buy the toxic products noted in this book.

Send money to the organizations listed below that are trying to get the scientific proof to protect us. Knowledge is power. No matter what our congress does, no matter how much false information comes out from big chemical, big food and big pharm, we get to vote with what we buy. Get involved. 'Become **an army of one**.'

Join me.

ORGANIZATIONS TO FOLLOW AND SUPPORT

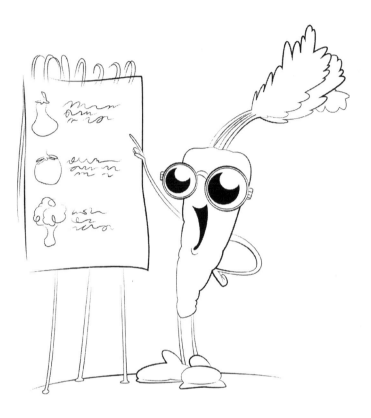

- **EWG.org**

EWG has a data base with hundreds of thousands of products and rates them on a toxicity scale of 1-10.

I have listed many of the products by category that I have found and now use in my life. It can be a bit daunting to use the data base, but the rewards are a healthier life.

EWG publishes the Dirty Dozen and The Clean 15 every year. If you can't buy all your fruits and vegies organic, these lists are a perfect place to start.

They have a **SKIN DEEP** data base for cosmetics and skin care. It never occurred to me that my head was itchy from toxic shampoos. My skin burned from most sunscreens, not the sun, but the sunscreen itself. Perfumes created breathing issues for me. Now I use healthy products.

They just finished breaking down thousands of **can goods**. My rule is if a food has something in it I can't pronounce I don't eat it. This data base can tell you what all those ingredients to do you.

Take time to peruse this site. It is a gold mine of information. It will make your life a whole lot more comfortable. If you are struggling with inflammation, it will help you eliminate the toxic chemicals that surround you.

Moms Across America
I now follow Moms Across America on Facebook. Started by a Mom, Zen Honeycutt, who *wants* to protect her children from Monsanto, Bayer, and other pesticide and herbicides being sprayed on our food and causing HUGE health issues, first in our children, and now in our adults. This is a great place to learn about the corruption in growing our foods. They have a testimonial tab; take a look at Mom's success stories with their children when toxins are removed from their children's foods. They are also involved with the whole vaccination issue and with how we are being gouged by the Pharmaceutical companies. This is a must organization for every Mom. Zen is an amazing **"Army of One."**

- **Organic Consumers Organization**
Another activist group trying to protect us from being poisoned. They are part of the fight to label GMOs.

- **The Cornucopia Institute**
Another group doing vast research on the effects of chemicals on our environment, our bodies, our children, our lives. They are doing research on all of the toxic chemicals in our lives and on GMOs.

All four of these organizations are doing tremendous work on our behalf to uncover all of the toxins being used in our food and supplies and all four are trying to stop the pollution of our crops, our products, our foods, our lives.

The first stage is awareness of what is happening. The second stage is to support the crusaders who want to stop the corruption and want to stop corporations from poisoning us.

- **Robyn O'Brien**

A call out as well to Robyn O'Brien, Another Mom who was astonished at what is being allowed by our Pharmaceuticals and our food. She is the Erin Brockovich of food and drugs. Watch her UTubes, and follow her on Facebook. She is amazing. She got involved to save our children. She truly is "**An Army of One.**"

Where to do at home testing for food Sensitivities

- **Everly Well**

This company is fairly new, and they offer at home tests that you send in to get food sensitivities. I had my test done with my doctor, but in lieu of that, this could be a great place to start.

Movies

I joined <u>Food Matters</u>, and they have a remarkable library of Movies on Health as well as fabulous recipes, and other Healthy tips

Movies that will change your awareness

- Vaxxed
- Origins
- Fat, Sick and Nearly Dead
- The Truth About Cancer
- Fed Up
- Genetic Roulette
- Tons of Movies on Food Matters.com http://www.foodmatters.com/films

Books

My favorite book is Dr. Libby Weaver's book **Accidentally Overweight** Hay House, Inc.; 1 edition (March 1, 2016).

This book is valuable to all, with or without a weight problem. She is a PHD Biochemist and goes body system by body system. She starts with what to know if it is not working properly, and then has an action plan at the end of each chapter. Her premise is that the entire body has to work properly to reach your ideal weight and optimal health. Since I have been eating clean now for 3 years, and am still struggling with weight (I have lost 45 pounds and still have 40 to go) her premise makes sense.

Chapter 28

Amazing people who are leading the way, educating us and taking on the system

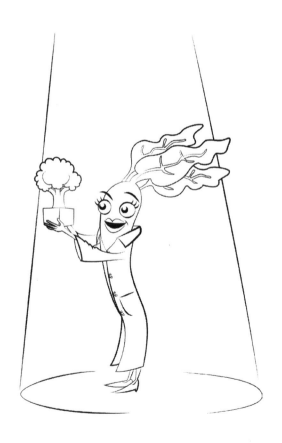

MY GOLDEN BROCCOLI AWARD GOES TO….

Functional Doctors to follow

- Mark Hyman, MD – leader in the Functional Medicine Movement. On the Board for the Institute for Functional Medicine
  http://drhyman.com/
- Amy Myers, MD – Autoimmune disease, Thyroid Disease, has a remote program with support for autoimmune disease. Contact her team in Austin, TX. Has a fabulous book on autoimmune disease which you should read. Great information on her website. Follow her for additional information weekly. She and her staff offer a remote support program for people suffering with autoimmune disease.
  http://www.amymyersmd.com/
- Daniel Amen, MD – The Brain Doctor/ Wife is a Nutritionist and RN. His brain school is amazing and everything you need to protect yourself from Brain disorders in old age. Become a brain warrior. His wife Tara is a nutritionist and an amazing inspiration as well.
  http://www.amenclinics.com/
- Josh Axe, ND – Informative blogs on a variety of subjects in the quest for wellness One of the first places I look for information.
  https://draxe.com/
- Tom O'Bryan DC, CCN, DACBN – Concentrates on Gluten diseases and Autoimmune Disease He also directed and produced the movie "***Betrayed***" about how conventional medicine is failing to confront and treat autoimmune disease. Has an amazing book on autoimmune disease which you should read. **The Autoimmune Fix** Dr. Tom O'Bryan Rodale Books; 1st edition
  http://certifiedglutenpractitioner.com/
- Susan Blum, Functional MD – an early practitioner of functional medicine. She does programs United States wide from her clinic in NY, with phone and Skype support. She has an incredible book out on autoimmune disease, which you should read. **The Immune System Recovery Plan: A Doctor's 4-Step Program to Treat Autoimmune Disease** Dr. Susan Blum, MD Scribner; 1st edition (April 2, 2013)
  http://blumcenterforhealth.com/functional-medicine/
- Suzy Cohen RPh – Functional Medicine practitioner and Registered

Pharmacist, Amazing blog, great supplements, her book **Drug Muggers** Rodale Books; 1ˢᵗ edition (February 15, 2011) is a must. She has been the first person I read to discuss many issues that I am now pursuing with my functional MD.
http://suzycohen.com/

- Tieraona Low Dog, MD – A herbalist, a MD, Spirit Walker, American Indian wisdom and philosophy
  https://drlowdog.com/

- Aviva Romm, MD – herbalist and midwife, amazing information for health, with an emphasis on women's issues and hormones. Great blogs
  https://avivaromm.com/

- Dr. Russell Blaylock, MD – I subscribed his newsletter for 15 years. He is a neurologist that lost both his parents to Parkinson's, and started looking for a better way to serve his patients. Things that I am reading frequently now by the functional community were ideas discussed in Dr. Blaylock's newsletters years ago.
  http://blaylockreport.com/

- Frank Lipman, MD – Detoxing, functional eating for health. I love his Sunday morning *Be Well Blog*, always informative.
  https://www.bewell.com/blog/

- David Perlmutter, MD – a board-certified neurologist and a Fellow of the American College of Nutrition Brain-Gut Connection Neurology He does amazing interviews with Functional Doctors and researchers
  http://www.drperlmutter.com/

- Dr. Joseph Mercola, DO – writes thought provoking articles and often covers subjects long before other people that I follow. A must to follow and to stay informed.
  http://www.mercola.com/

- Vikki Peterson, DC, CCN, CFMP – a ND, Vegan, great cooking videos and blogs on the benefits of vegan living
  http://healthnowmedical.com/

- Brian Mowll, ND – http://drbrianmowll.com/ fields of expertise Diabetes, essential oils
  http://drbrianmowll.com/

- Emeran Mayers, MD – executive director of the UCLA Oppenheimer Center for the Neurobiology of Stress, **Brain – Gut Connection**

http://emeranmayer.com/
- Joel Kahn, MD – Heart Doctor/ Vegan strong advice for heart issues
  https://drjoelkahn.com/
- Jennifer Fugo, CRT – Health Coach Owns the Gluten Free School. Essential information for anyone struggling with Gluten issues.
  http://www.evolvingwell.com/
- JJ Virgin, CNS, CHFS – The Sugar Guru
  http://jjvirgin.com/
- Sara Wilson – of **I Quit Sugar**, another sugar guru.
  http://www.sarahwilson.com/
- Sean Croxton – Health interviewer (great pod casts) on U Tube, shifting now to Personal Growth. A wonderful daily Inspiration, 3 minutes long. A great way to start the day
  http://seancroxton.com/
- Jeffry Smith – the Founder and Executive Director of the Institute for Responsible Technology is running the Campaign for Healthier Eating in America -leading the way to inform us on the dangers of GMO's
  http://responsibletechnology.org/
- Wendy Myers, FDN-P, NC, CHHC – her field of practice is Heavy Toxic Metals. Get on her newsletter list. Get informed. She has a guide for all the toxic metals and what they could be doing in your body.
  https://liveto110.com/
- Dr. Ben Lynch – a licensed naturopathic physician specializing in **MTHFR** mutations, epigenetics and clinical ecology, my go to guru on Methylation. The science involving Methylation is constantly being updated. I try to catch a new interview with Dr. Lynch each month and always learn something new I can use.
  www.drbenlynch.com
- Ocean Robbins – environmentalist, working to save the planet to save us all
  http://oceanrobbins.com/
- Dr. Deanna Minich – a functional Dr. of Nutrition, is a proponent of eating all the colors of the rainbow, and an expert on detox.
  http://deannaminich.com/
- Dr. Libby Weaver– PhD, biochemist with an expertise in nutrition. Looks at the entire body and how it functions together. Brilliant and easy to read. In my next life, I want to be a biochemist like Dr. Libby. Her **Accidentally**

Overweight book Hay House, Inc.; 1 edition (March 1, 2016) is essential for anyone dealing with health issues to understand how the entire body has to work in unison to create wellness. For the first time, I started to see the big picture from her book. Not only for people with weight issues, and ideal for anyone with Autoimmune Disease.
https://www.drlibby.com/

Chapter 29

Professionals critical to my wellness journey

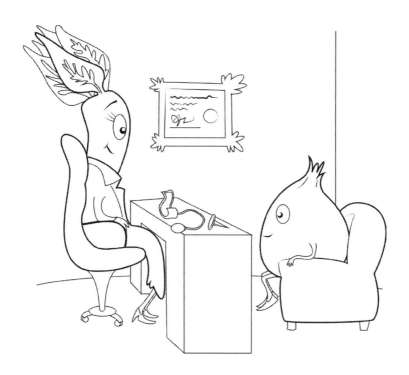

331

MY WIZARDS OF HEALTH

MY FUNCTIONAL MD

- **Shilpa Sayana, MD**
  Studio City, California Sayana Medical Integrative Care
  818-331-4386
  https://www.sayanamedical.com/shilpa-sayana-md

I was super sick when I became a patient of Dr. Sayana. She listened to me, asked questions no previous doctor had ever asked, and we are working on issues that my body has one by one. She is an amazing doctor. She is uncovering many root causes for my inflammation, one by one, like peeling an onion. Currently not accepting any other new patients, she does have an ND and a Nurse Practitioner, both certified in Functional Medicine in her office. She is currently looking for additional Functional Practitioners. Her office accepts insurance. She has an associate that is specializing in children. Dr. Sayana is a doctor practicing compassionate functional medicine.

- **Susan Spizer, LAc**
  suespizer1@me.com
  A member of Dr. Sayana's team
  https://www.sayanamedical.com/susan-spizer-lac

Sue is trained in Frequency Specific Microcurrent, which has reduced my pain dramatically. She is also certified by the Institute of Functional Medicine, and is very knowledgeable at helping find root causes for inflammation. I did my initial liver detoxes with her, and tested for pesticide in my system with Sue, which I am now detoxing out of my system with Dr. Sayana. Amazing health provider. Compassionate and caring

- **Destiny Saenz**
  Masseuse, Los Angeles Area, California
  d_saenz@msn.com – 818-384-3094

Destiny is amazing with gifted healing hands. She will travel and do massages in your home. I have been going to her for almost 10 years and she has worked wonders with stiff and annoyed muscles and cramps.

BIOLOGICAL DENTIST

- **LA Holistic Dentistry**
  10850 Wilshire Blvd Ste 330, Los Angeles
  http://drrota.com/ – 310-208-4297

Dr. Rota, the original dentist at this practice is the mastermind that developed Biological Dentistry to remove toxic mercury fillings back in the 1980's when he was at UCLA. He recently retired, but he fully trained the dentists that now own his practice.

Getting my fillings removed was like a scene from a science fiction novel. Their procedure fully protected me from both the fumes of the mercury metal and from the fragments going into my system. This was the first step in metal detoxification. I was not able to begin the detox of mercury until my fillings were removed, because the detox would have pulled more mercury into my system. The procedure was very cutting edge and totally worth it. With the detox itself that followed the removal of my amalgams, I am now mercury free. Highly recommended. If you are not in Los Angeles, search for a Biological dentist in your area.

- **Body and Brain**
  Scott and Junie Lee
  120 W Lemon Ave, Monrovia, CA 91016 – 626 386-5300

An awesome facility for Korean Dao Yoga, a gentle form of movement, resistance and stretching exercise that I, who hate to exercise, have learned to love. It also appeals to my spiritual self. I am also grateful for the community of really cool people that exercise there.

Body and Brain is a National group with facilities across the country. We also enjoyed a fabulous weekend at their Sedona Retreat in Arizona, which was good for the soul in a very beautiful location, with delicious Pescatarian food and very wise sages.

Chapter 30

How to become an agent of change, an army of one

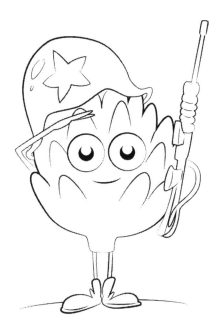

In this book, I share an enormous amount of information on toxins, how they are destroying your health and the health of your family and how to replace those products in your life.

I also share how our government is not protecting us. I was hoping that measures would be passed protecting us from GMOs, and when that did not happen, it occurred to me, we can vote with our dollars and change the system that way. Our elected officials aren't going to help us. There is just too much money, honey.

I have read that it will only take a 5% change in our spending habits to have Big Food, and Big Pharma pay attention and then they will start to change. It has started, but we need to join together to make sure it happens more quickly.

We each have the ability to make better decisions for our lives and for our families. I am asking you to be an agent of change, and to become an army of one.

1. Spread the word.

2. Join the movement.

3. If you are a parent, join Moms Across America.

4. Vote with every product you purchase.

5. Call your congressman and senator often and demand cleaner air, cleaner water, that we ban toxins in our food and label GMOs, control Big Pharm from price gouging when it comes to our children. Don't call once, call often. Be active. We don't have to take it anymore. Make yourself heard.

6. Support EWG, The Organic Consumers organization, Cornucopia or other fine organizations that are working on our behalf to educate us and fight for our health.

7. Knowledge is power. We need to support these organizations to keep us informed.

8. Purge the toxic substances from your life, one by one, until they are gone.

9. Follow the doctors and other experts that I list for constant updates that will impact your health. Go to their website and join to receive their newsletters.

10. Share your knowledge, but each of us gets to decide for ourselves what to do. You can change what you do, and be the change you want to see. You can be the example.

11. Educate your children to make better choices. Their lives depend on it.

Part 7

What we've learned, What comes next

What we've learned, what comes next,
become a member of my tribe

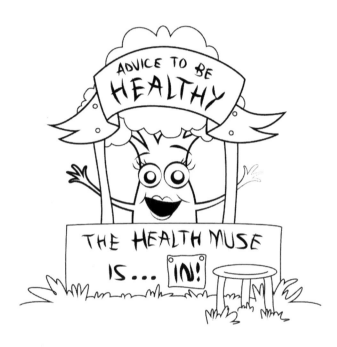

FOR A QUICK RECAP OF WHAT YOU HAVE LEARNED
IN THIS BOOK, REFER BACK TO THE INITIAL CHAPTER
CALLED DEDICATION, HOW TO USE THIS BOOK.

WITH LITTLE STEPS, EACH DAY, WE CAN EACH TAKE
BACK OUR OWN HEALTH AND *BECOME AN ARMY OF*
ONE. JOIN ME, AND LET'S GO CHANGE THE WORLD!

FREE EBOOK WORKBOOK

Contact me at cherylmhealthmuse@gmail.com for a **free workbook to download.** It will help you organize what steps you choose to take first, and stay focused so that you can accomplish them. Highly recommended.

LIKE ME ON FACEBOOK

My page is cherylmhealthmuse. Information changes daily and my toxic database is being constantly updated. I post articles that I think are most relevant to your health and the health of your families.

SIGN UP FOR MY NEWSLETTERS

There is a pop-up sign up for my newsletter button when you log on to htttp://cherylmhealthmuse.com. My newsletters are filled with wonderful ideas to promote your health and will keep you up-to-date with new information and new offerings.

WHAT IS COMING NEXT

If you follow me, you will be the first to know about my future releases geared towards your health. My next project is three-fold:

1. How to eat organic on a budget.

2. How to make quick and healthy meals at home.

3. All the tricks that I have learned to live this way. It's fun and I am not deprived. I want to share these tips with you.

Need more help? Hire me as your health coach. Contact me for a free 1 hour consultation and I can provide you the details.

PRIVATE COACHING

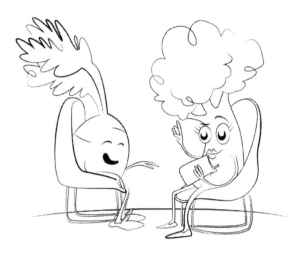

If you want to adopt the strategies in this book, but need more guidance, I am available for individual health coaching or as I called it in the book, the private guided tour. Contact me through my website, cherylmhealthmuse.com or at cherylmhealthmuse@gmail.com.

I have different packages available. We all have busy lives, so I offer packages with flexible timeframes that will work best with your busy life.

- An hour to sort out how to move forward
- A package of 6 one hour sessions, to use and work with me over a 4-month period, with flexibility to guide you in the getting started phase.
- A package of 12 hours enough to help you realize sustainable change. This is a package with flexible times over an 8-month period.
- A design it yourself program. I am here to help you create the support and the wellness you deserve.

GROUP COACHING ON INFLAMMATION AND TOXINS (TO COME, DATES TO BE ANNOUNCED)

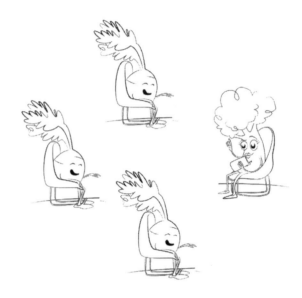

The group guided tour – I will be developing programs where I literally am the tour guide to a group with pain and inflammation issues. These will be designed for more people at an affordable cost than the private coaching packages and will include a private Facebook page and office hours once a month.

This could be live group coaching, web group coaching or webinars in the future, so sign up now for my newsletter and don't miss out.

HIRE ME TO SPEAK TO YOUR GROUP

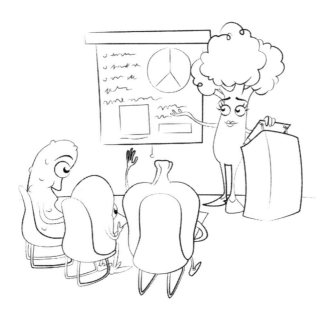

Specialties are

- Eliminating toxins from your world.
- Reversing inflammation.
- How I live with food and toxin restrictions including, shopping, travel, eating out, eating at other's homes, how to make better choices, how to do this and not that. Eating organic on a budget. Cooking healthy food at home as a quick order chef. I am not deprived and can help others figure this out too. It's fun and rewarding.
- Toxic minds, stress, *ants*, movement, relationships and how they impact wellness.
- Diabetes (like inflammation, it can be reversed with lifestyle changes.)
- Detoxing.

CONTACT ME

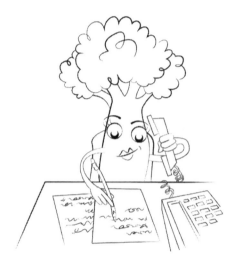

I would love you to contact me with your health concerns. It will help me target and communicate the right information in my newsletter and on face book. cherylmhealthmuse@gmail.com

No matter what, KEEP GOING. You will learn how great it is, to feel good again, and it will all be worth it.

HOW TO BECOME A HEALTH COACH/ANOTHER WAY TO BE AN ARMY OF ONE/THE RIPPLE EFFECT

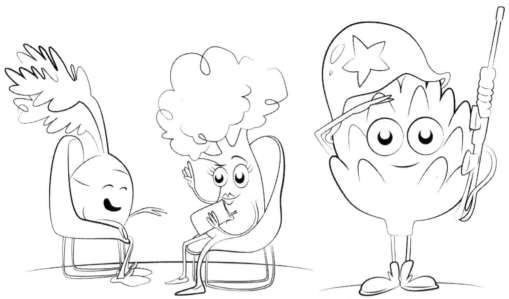

This book was inspired by my experience at the Institute for Integrative Nutrition® (IIN), where I received my training as a holistic wellness and health coach. I also took their "Launch Your Own Dream Book" course, which guided me in writing this book.

IIN offers a truly comprehensive Health Coach Training Program that invites students to deeply explore the things that are most nourishing to them. From the physical aspects of nutrition and eating wholesome foods that work best for each individual person, to the concept of Primary Food – the idea that everything in life, including our spirituality, career, relationships, and fitness contributes to our inner and outer health – IIN helped me reach optimal health and balance.

I set out on a journey to heal my pain and inflammation 5 years ago and in the last year, IIN gave me the certification to share what I have learned. I am quite passionate about my journey and I want to help and inspire others.

We are a sick nation, and we are getting sicker. This is an emerging field for a fulfilling career. If you are inspired by what you have learned in my book and want to join the movement, taking the 1 year online course from IIN is a perfect way to start. What you learn will enhance your own personal journey to wellness and in addition, will teach you health coaching, as well as the business and marketing needed to run your own health coaching business.

Students who choose to pursue this field professionally complete the program equipped with the communication skills and branding knowledge they need to create a fulfilling career encouraging and supporting others in reaching their own health goals.

Students embark in many different directions upon graduation, and each has their own unique focus. I want to help others identify inflammation, and then make lifestyle changes to reverse the disease. I have also become an advocate that we must vote with our dollars if we want to eliminate the toxins in our world.

Others want to work with moms with limited time and children, and/or work to improve food in the school system; some want to work with people with Thyroid conditions. Some ... become organic chefs and train others how to cook for health. You can use this education in your own unique way once you graduate. There are dozens of ways to use this knowledge to make a difference in the world.

From renowned wellness experts as Visiting Teachers to the convenience of their online learning platform, this school has changed my life, and I believe it will do the same for you. I invite you to learn more about the Institute for Integrative Nutrition and explore how the Health Coach Training Program can help you transform your life. Feel free to contact me to hear more about my personal experience at www. cherylmhealthmuse.com/integrativenutrition. Or call (844) 315-8546 to learn more. Tell them Cheryl Meyer, the Health Muse, sent you!

Acknowledgements

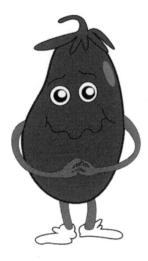

First and foremost, I am so grateful to my husband of 2 years, **John Gins**. What a remarkable partner he is. John embraces all of me, the good, the bad and the, well, if not ugly, certainly the different … and is always supportive. He set out on this journey with me 5 years ago to support me to find wellness. Along the way, he has lost 70 pounds and considers himself my first coaching success story.

For this book, John has been my sounding board. He has done additional reading when I got bogged down in the writing process. He has read some chapters 20 times and become my punctuation, grammar and content police. As a statistician and computer phenome, he formatted the book, moved the endnotes from the bottom of separate chapters, to the back of the book, and did the index (all of which were tasks that I would have twitched over.) He remained cheerful when I didn't have it in me to make dinner, and moved to the kitchen to cook. He never complained when I had my warmup naps at night watching TV before bed after writing for 14 hours. This book would not exist without his support and love, and I thank him from the bottom of my heart. I am one very lucky girl! I love him, and he makes me happy.

To **Nicholas Patton**, illustrator extraordinaire, for the truly amazing illustrations he did to add a touch of humor to very dry material. He is so gifted and I am so lucky to have his illustrations in my book. No one could have done it better.

Next, a big call out to **Scott Lee**, who owns the **Body and Brain** Korean Yoga studio in Monrovia, CA where we exercise. Scott took the manuscript, and as a former Aerospace engineer, edited my book with scientist's eye and a fine-tooth comb. What a gift Scott is to John and I and we are blessed to have him in our life. And to boot, he has encouraged me to find joy in movement and he and his wife, Junie have been a big part of my wellness success.

Val Peterson- my long-distance friend for 15 years that I have never met. Val and I became pen pals when she discovered me through my jewelry design on a shopping channel show. (My previous profession.) She has been an important part of my life now, weekly, for all these years through the beauty of Facebook messenger service. Val took my manuscript, read it carefully, and then started to implement my suggestions at rocket speed. As a result of her desire to follow my advice, I almost created world war III at her house when she threw out many of her husband's favorite foods. (Hence, the chapter at the beginning of my book, "How to Use This Book.") *smile* This story has a happy ending. Val and I came up with compromises she suggested to her hubby doing a **Do This, Not That Strategy**, and he got on board quickly in what is now their combined pursuit for optimal wellness. I learned a lot, as Val gave me feedback, and I am very grateful to have her in my life.

Other people that deserve a call out:

Jeanne Orfinik, my dear friend of 40 years, with a background in journalism, read the first chapter, made much appreciated suggestions, and got my writing on track.

Susan Qinghua Shi, my trusted sidekick, who returned from China last Dec to run my jewelry business through the holiday season, allowing me to concentrate on writing.

Jane Ho and **Queenie Li**, who do their jobs in my jewelry business with no supervision now, so that I can pursue a new career as a holistic health coach and share my office with both businesses. They are the best!

Destiny Saenz, one of my two initial clients, and also my remarkable masseuse, both for what I am learning in encouraging her to a healthier life as one of my first clients, and also for working all of the knots out of my body for sitting in one place at the computer for days and months on end writing this book. I have enjoyed her magic hands now for over 10 years. (Her business is **The Magic Hour**, and it is appropriately named.) She has remarkably gifted hands.

To **Cheryl Barron**, my other initial client, for everything I am learning in our sessions together.

To my Functional Medicine team, **Dr. Shilpa Sayana**, MD and **Sue Spizer** MTCM, LAc., for saving my life, reversing my inflammation and quelling my pain. And I thank them for their incredible knowledge, and dedication to my healing and guidance and for allowing me to be an active participant in my own health. They just keep digging deeper to heal me from the many weirdnesses in my health. A call out as well, to the rest of her team, for becoming like family, **Lara, Niza**, and **Sami**, encouraging me along this path. I am very grateful for their compassionate gift of healing. I am also grateful for their support as I embark on my new adventure to help others with what I have learned.

I am also very grateful for my friend **Elizabeth Brimmer**, for her continual support; **Kirsten Larsen,** for being an awesome accountability coach for this book; **Susie Begam-Violette**, for being a sounding board on the new paradigm of medicine, and **Barbara Lunger** for suggesting illustrations as a way to lighten my content.

To **Kim Hodges**, my health coach, for her guidance in my journey towards health.

To **Dr. Tony Ganem**, DC, where I began my journey, for being honest with me that I was a very sick girl. This made me regroup and take responsibility for my own health. And I am grateful for everything that I learned from him back in the beginning, and I appreciate his patience. Everything he was sharing was like I was listening to a foreign language that I didn't speak. I wish I had a picture of the look on my face as he was explaining things that in retrospect became clearer and clearer as I continued my journey.

To **Suzy Cohen**, RPh Author of "Drug Muggers: Which Medications Are Robbing Your Body of Essential Nutrients and How to Restore Them." **Rodale Books**; 1st edition (February 15, 2011) who responded with such support when I asked for permission to quote her, I was overwhelmed. Suzy writes blogs that have often had cutting edge information that I needed to peel additional layers off my onion in search of my health. She sent me her latest book **"Thyroid Healthy, Lose Weight, Look Beautiful and Live the Life You Imagine"** Dear Pharmacist Inc.; 1st edition (April 22, 2014) and volunteered to write a quote for the back of my book. Wow, Suzy, you are the best! I also use many of her supplements, with confidence in their quality. She also offered incredible support promoting this book.

To the other functional doctors who have allowed me to quote them in my book. **Dr. Mark Hyman**, MD, **Dr. Josh Axe**, ND, **Dr. Daniel Amen**, MD, **Dr. Joseph Mercola**, DO, **Dr. Frank Lipman**, MD, **Dr. Russell Blaylock** MD, (who was the first of the bunch that I started to follow), **Dr. David Jockers, Ocean Robbins** and **John Robbins** of the Baskin Robbins family, each an environmentalist in their own right, **Dr. Tieraona Low Dog**, MD, **Dr. Andrew Weil**, MD, and **Dr. Aviva Romm**, MD. I follow your blogs, your Facebook posts and read your books. Thank you so much for the continuing perspective and great information.

A special call out to **Dr. Susan Blum**, MD who took the time to write to me to ensure I understood the mechanism of leaky gut, and to **Sara Jennings**, from the Institute For Responsible Technology, who wrote and called me to explain further what GMOs actually were. (I had them confused with conventional farming ... and both use disgusting chemicals).

To Dr. Amy Myers, MD, Dr. Tom O'Bryan, DC CCN, DACBN, Dr. Libby Weaver, PhD, Sarah Wilson, JJ Virgin, CNS, CHFS, Sean Croxton, Dr. Joel Kahn, MD (heart specialist), Vikki Peterson, DC, CCN, CFMP, ND, Jennifer Fugo, CRT, Deanna Minich, PhD, FACN, CNS, Brian Mowll, ND, Dr. David Perlmutter, MD, Emeran Myers, MD, Wendy Myers, FDN-P, NC, CHHP, and Food Matters, whose books I devoured and webinars I devoted myself to like a sponge to learn to heal myself.

To **Dr. Ben Lynch**, ND for his research and promotion of the perils of the Methylation anomaly on our DNA. I follow you to understand my own methylation issue, along with my doctors' guidance.

To **Terry Wahls**, MD for her inspirational story of reversing her debilitating MS and gaining her life back. She gave me hope.

To EWG, The Cornucopia Institute, The Organic Consumers Association, and The Institute for Responsible Technology, for continuing to do the research and keep us informed about all of the toxins in our lives.

To **Robyn O'Brien** children's health advocate, and **Zen Honeycutt**, Founder and Executive Director, **Moms Across America**, for your research and for fighting for all of us for a healthier tomorrow. You are the true Armies of One that we need to join.

JOIN THEM AND VOTE WITH YOUR DOLLARS.

Thank you to all of the doctors and partici*pants* of the following symposiums that I devoured trying to help myself get well.

- The Detox Summit
- The Supplement Summit
- **Sean Croxton**, The Second Opinion Series, Digestion, Thyroid, Depression
- The Hashimotos Summit
- The Fat Summit 2
- The Sleep Summit
- The Diabetes Summit, 1, 2, and 3
- The Thyroid Connection
- The Healing Leaky Gut Program
- The Gluten Free School Forum
- The Autoimmune Summit
- Holistic Oral Health
- Alzheimer's Dementia Summit
- The Total Wellness Summit
- The Truth About Cancer
- Betrayal, how the current medical system is failing those of us with Autoimmune Disease.

Kris Carr and her Meditations, soothing me from her gentle and kind soul.

These are all summits that were given for free by health professionals that had joined the functional community to heal themselves from disease and then wanted to help others. What a gift you all are. I love what I learned so much, I bought each of the summits and have the information to refer back to. Because of you, I too want to give back.

To the patient, kind and knowledgeable team at The Institute Of Integrative Nutrition® "Launch Your Own Book" course. Thanks to all, and especially to **Sue Brown** and **Liz Palmieri** for the continual support and amazing creativity to help all of us hatch our books. Thank you as well, **Joshua Rosenthal**, Founder and Director of IIN®.

And finally, but certainly not least, I am so grateful to my parents, **Edith and George Hunsinger**. My joke with my Mom was that I chose my parents really well before I was born. She used to chuckle and say I must have been hatched, because no daughter of hers would say such a thing. *smile*

I DID pick well, and thank them for their unconditional love and for their encouragement that I was a Hunsinger (my maiden name) and that I could do anything I set my mind to. What a remarkable gift. Both of my parents suffered from unusual illnesses. Both took medications that became as big an issue as their disease was. I wish I knew then, what I know now. I could have, perhaps, helped them find the help and relief that they so sorely needed.

Thank you for allowing me to share my gratitude for all of the remarkable people who have touched my life and lent me support in this project. It brings me joy. I believe it is important to show gratitude on a daily basis as part of a healthy mind and healthy body.

Index

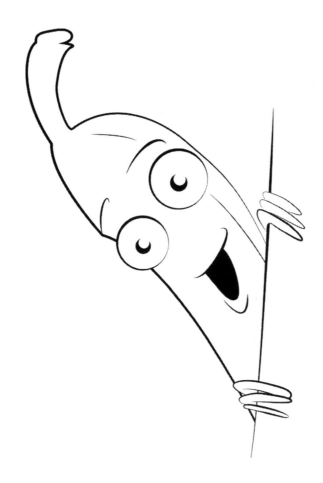

W

End Notes

DEDICATION

2 Pegan is a term coined by Mark Hyman, MD. It is a great way to eat organic pastured meat, and still stay on a budget.

3 You can find a Functional Practitioner by going to the Institute for Functional Medicine and putting in your zip code. I travel 1 hour to see my functional MD. One of the best decisions I have made ever. https://www.functionalmedicine.org/practitioner_search.aspx?id=117

INTRODUCTION

5 Words I use most often on Facebook

6 Read Dr. Libby Weavers book "Accidentally Overweight." Hay House, Inc.; 1 edition (March 1, 2016) It's the first explanation that I found that explained how our bodies work and that if everything is not "in tune," it's practically impossible to release the toxic weight.

7 "The Paleo Diet- from Wikipedia, "the diet typically includes vegetables, fruits, nuts, roots, meat, and organ meats and fish while excluding foods such as dairy products, grains, sugar, legumes, processed oils, salt, and alcohol or coffee." I eat a modified version of this diet. I still eat beans, which the Paleo diet does not include. Beans are not foods that were available to cavemen. I use nut flours in the place of grains. We do eat some rice and quinoa. I still occasionally drink coffee. I eliminated alcohol because it conflicted with an organic compounded thyroid I am taking.
Vegetarian or Vegan diets may work better for you.
Vegetarian Diet- from Wikipedia, "is the practice of abstaining from the consumption of meat (red meat, poultry, seafood, and the flesh of any other animal), and may also include abstention from by-products of animal slaughter.

8

9 Diet- from Wikipedia "is both the practice of abstaining from the use of animal products, particularly in diet" Pronounced "VEEGAN."

10 Raw Diet –Raw means you don't cook your food. Food is not cooked above 118° so that you get maximum nutrients from the food. Raw is a more restrictive version of Vegan. If you decide to follow the raw approach and choose to include meat and fish, the meat and fish are cooked. (and clean, to be discussed further).

11 https://www.ewg.org/foodnews/dirty_dozen_list.php

CHAPTER 1 WHAT IS A HEALTH COACH AND WHY DID I BECOME ONE?

13 *ANTs* is a term coined by Daniel Amen MD and stands for "Anxious Negative Thoughts

14 A term coined by Daniel Amen, MD

15 http://simplereminders.com/quotes/sometimes-smallest-step-must-take-step.html

16 http://mastinkipp.com/

CHAPTER 2 YOU CAN'T CHANGE WHAT YOU DON'T UNDERSTAND- INFLAMMATION

18 Already Always Listening™ Landmark Worldwide, LLC. http://www.trademarkia.com/map/already-always-listening-78113582.html

19 Somewhere in my retail management training over *20* years ago, I learned this term and dearly love it. I have searched for its origin, to no avail.

20 http://tinybuddha.com/wisdom-quotes/given-moment-power-say-story-going-end/

21 Already Always Listening™ Landmark Worldwide, LLC. http://www.trademarkia.com/map/already-always-listening-78113582.html

22 http://www.goodreads.com/quotes/*424358*-don-t-believe-everything-you-think-thoughts-are-just-that--

CHAPTER 3 WHAT IS THE FUNCTIONAL MEDICINE APPROACH?

24 *The Immune System Recovery Plan: A Doctor's 4-Step Program to Treat Autoimmune Disease Dr. Susan Blum, MD* Scribner; *1* edition (April *2, 2013*)

25 https://www.functionalmedicine.org/what_is_functional_medicine/aboutfm/

26 *The Immune System Recovery Plan: A Doctor's 4-Step Program to Treat Autoimmune Disease Dr. Susan Blum, MD* Scribner; *1* edition (April *2, 2013*)

27 https://en.wikipedia.org/wiki/Miracle_on_34th_Street

28 https://www.functionalmedicine.org/practitioner_search.aspx?id=*117*

CHAPTER 4 WHAT IS AUTOIMMUNE DISEASE?

30 http://www.medicinenet.com/script/main/art.asp?articlekey=*2402*

31 http://www.amymyersmd.com/*2017/01*/part-i-*8*-truths-about-autoimmunity/

32 http://www.amymyersmd.com/*2017/01*/part-i-*8*-truths-about-autoimmunity/

33 Dr. Amy Myers *"5 Secrets About Autoimmunity"* webinar *2/20/17*

34 Dr. Amy Myers *"5 Secrets About Autoimmunity"* webinar *2/20/17*

35 Dr. Amy Myers *"5 Secrets About Autoimmunity"* webinar *2/20/17*

[36] *The Immune System Recovery Plan: A Doctor's 4-Step Program to Treat Autoimmune Disease* **Dr. Susan Blum, MD** Scribner; 1 edition (April 2, 2013)

[37] http://solvingleakygut.com/drtom/

[38] *The Immune System Recovery Plan: A Doctor's 4-Step Program to Treat Autoimmune Disease* **Dr. Susan Blum, MD** Scribner; 1 edition (April 2, 2013)

[39] *The Autoimmune Solution: Prevent and Reverse the Full Spectrum of Inflammatory Symptoms and Diseases* **Dr. Amy Myers, MD** HarperOne; 1 edition (January 27, 2015)

[40] http://solvingleakygut.com/drtom/

[41] Dr. Amy Myers "5 Secrets About Autoimmunity" webinar 2/20/17

[42] Dr. Amy Myers "5 Secrets About Autoimmunity" webinar 2/20/17

[43] Dr. Amy Myers "5 Secrets About Autoimmunity" webinar 2/20/17

[44] *The Immune System Recovery Plan: A Doctor's 4-Step Program to Treat Autoimmune Disease* **Dr. Susan Blum, MD** Scribner; 1 edition (April 2, 2013)

[45] Susan Blum, MD via email on the effects of sugar on the gut 1/27/17

[46] Susan Blum, MD via email on best oils to heal autoimmune disease 1/27/17

[47] http://solvingleakygut.com/drtom/

CHAPTER 5 ONE LAST THOUGHT – FLARES

[49] A flare refers to a set of unexpected reactions to environmental changes in your body.

INTRODUCTION CLEANING UP THE TOXINS IN YOUR LIFE.

[51] http://www.nejm.org/doi/full/10.1056/NEJMp0910064

[52] I was introduced to Howard Lyman in a lecture at IIN©. I heard his call, and strive to be "an army of one"

[53] http://www.bing.com/images/search?q=absence+of+evidence+quote&view=detailv2&&id=979A976825AB4A8EA529215F9025AE779DDD2F41&selectedIndex=0&ccid=ZNyF6ULc&simid=608007816714782761&thid=OIP.ZNyF6ULcVDmqrG2SwZakdwEhEh&ajaxhist=0

[54] http://www.argentinaindependent.com/currentaffairs/latest-news/newsfromargentina/professor-denounces-persecution-after-testifying-at-monsanto-tribunal/

[55] Howard Lyman **No More Bull** Scribner (September 20, 2005) available on Amazon

[56] http://www.urbandictionary.com/define.php?term=Army%20of%20One

[57] http://www.all-creatures.org/articles/mdi-nature-not-negotiate.html

[58] "**The Telomere Effect: A Revolutionary Approach to Living Younger, Healthier, Longer** by Dr. Elizabeth Blackburn, Dr. Elissa Epel Grand Central Publishing (January 3, 2017)

PREFACE ORDER THE DUMPSTER; THERE ARE TOXINS TO PURGE

60 https://www.theburningplatform.com/2016/01/20/what-genius-thinks-of-education/
61 Food Matters http://store.foodmatters.com/?_ga=1.196868140.1893475740.1486086009
62 .ANTs is a term coined by Daniel Amen MD and stands for "Anxious Negative Thoughts."
63 ANTs is a term coined by Daniel Amen MD and stands for "Anxious Negative Thoughts
64 Dr. Tom O'Bryan The Autoimmune Fix Rodale Books; 1 edition (September 20, 2016)
65 Phrase used by Dr. Susan Blum, Functional MD and autoimmune expert.
66 http://www.sourcewatch.org/index.php/Pharmaceutical_industry
67 Food Matters http://store.foodmatters.com/?_ga=1.196868140.1893475740.1486086009
68 GreenWave | The Buckminster Fuller Institute www.bfi.org/ideaindex/projects/2015/greenwave
69 http://www.thespiralpathway.com/
70 ANTs is a term coined by Daniel Amen MD and stands for "Anxious Negative Thoughts

CHAPTER 6 ORGANIC VS GMOS VS CONVENTIONAL FARMING

72 http://gmwatch.org/news/latest-news/17483 2/27/17 Published in GM Watch, The 750 studies that GMO regulatory bodies often ignore.
73 Robyn O'Brien Facebook posting 2/27/17
74 https://en.wikipedia.org/wiki/Organic_farming
75 http://www.who.int/topics/food_genetically_modified/en/
76 http://www.hellawella.com/top-10-reasons-organic-food-is-so-expensive/4727
77 http://www.hellawella.com/top-10-reasons-organic-food-is-so-expensive/4727
78 http://www.foxnews.com/food-drink/2015/08/18/top-reasons-why-organic-food-is-so-expensive.html
79 http://www.foxnews.com/food-drink/2015/08/18/top-reasons-why-organic-food-is-so-expensive.html
80 http://www.fao.org/organicag/oa-faq/oa-faq5/en/
81 http://www.foxnews.com/food-drink/2015/08/18/top-reasons-why-organic-food-is-so-expensive.html
82 http://www.foxnews.com/food-drink/2015/08/18/top-reasons-why-organic-food-is-so-expensive.html
83 https://www.thebalance.com/how-much-does-organic-certification-cost-2538018
84 http://www.organicauthority.com/does-organic-produce-spoil-faster-than-conventional/
85 http://www.hellawella.com/top-10-reasons-organic-food-is-so-expensive/4727

[86] http://www.altmedrev.com/publications/*15/1/4*.pdf

[87] http://healthy-organics.com.au/

[88] *Genetic Roulette, The Gamble Of Our Lives Movie*

[89] http://www.slideshare.net/digitalreporter/the-documented-health-risks-of-genetically-engineered-foods-long-version slide *42*

[90] http://www.ewg.org/

[91] https://www.ewg.org/foodnews/dirty_dozen_list.php

[92] http://whatsonmyfood.org/food.jsp?food=PO

[93] http://whatsonmyfood.org/food.jsp?food=SS

[94]

[95] http://articles.mercola.com/sites/articles/archive/*2011/10/04*/healthy-foods-you-should-never-ever-eat.aspx#!

[96] *Genetic Roulette, The Gamble Of Our Lives Movie*

[97] Jeffry Smith statement in *Genetic Roulette, The Gamble Of Our Lives Movie*

[98] http://www.greenpeace.org/international/en/news/Blogs/makingwaves/eat-it-up-monsanto/blog/*39002*/

[99] http://www.theorganicprepper.ca/gmos-not-even-in-moderation-*02072013*

[100] http://www.monsanto.com/improvingagriculture/pages/organic-and-conventional-agriculture.aspx

[101] http://www.monsantoito.com/docs/RoundupQuikPRO_Label.pdf

[102] http://www.latimes.com/business/la-fi-roundup-cancer-*20170127*-story.html

[103] http://healthimpactnews.com/*2011*/the-dangers-of-roundup-ready-food/

[104] https://www.academia.edu/*5772865*/GLYPHOSATE_IT_BINDS_MINERALS_AND_CUTS_OFF_THE_PRODUCTION_OF_NEUROTRANSMITTERS_AND_HORMONES....A_VISUAL_CONNECTION_OF_THE_ROUTES_OF_DISEASES_AND_CANCER

[105] http://naturalnews.com/*040482*_glyphosate_Monsanto_detoxification.html

[106] http://www.slideshare.net/digitalreporter/the-documented-health-risks-of-genetically-engineered-foods-long-version slide *127*

[107] http://chemicalindustryarchives.org/dirtysecrets/annistonindepth/toxicity.asp

[108] http://www.theorganicprepper.ca/gmos-not-even-in-moderation-*02072013*

[109] https://www.youtube.com/watch?v=ovKw*6*YjqSfM

[110] http://www.collective-evolution.com/*2014/04/08/10*-scientific-studies-proving-gmos-can-be-harmful-to-human-health/

[111] https://chriskresser.com/are-gmos-safe/

[112] https://www.amazon.com/Genetic-Roulette-Gamble-Our-Lives/dp/B*0096*DP4CG/ref=sr_*1_1*?s=movies-tv&ie=UTF*8*&qid=*1485361453*&sr=*1-1*-spons&keywords=genetic+roulette&psc=*1*

[113] http://www.slideshare.net/digitalreporter/the-documented-health-risks-of-genetically-engineered-foods-long-version slide *8*

[114] http://www.slideshare.net/digitalreporter/the-documented-health-risks-of-genetically-engineered-foods-long-version

[115] http://www.sciencedirect.com/science/article/pii/S*0890623811000566*

116   Jeffry Smith statement in *Genetic Roulette, The Gamble Of Our Lives Movie*
117   http://www.slideshare.net/digitalreporter/the-documented-health-risks-of-genetical-ly-engineered-foods-long-version slide *48*
118   Netherwood et al, "Assessing the survival of transgenic plant DNA in the human gastrointestinal tract," *Nature Biotechnology 22 (2004)*: 2.
119   http://www.gmo-compass.org/eng/agri_biotechnology/breeding_aims/*146*.herbicide_resistant_crops.html
120   http://newsletters.newsmax.com/blaylock/issues/heal*0117*/blaylock_heal*0117_151*.pdf
121   http://newsletters.newsmax.com/blaylock/issues/heal*0117*/blaylock_heal*0117_151*.pdf
122   http://www.globalhealingcenter.com/natural-health/effects-of-pesticides/
123   https://mail.google.com/mail/u/0/#inbox/*15989e5b28342b7a*
       http://www.monsanto.com/improvingagriculture/pages/organic-and-conventional-agriculture.aspx
       Increased food production
124   http://www.gmwatch.org/news/archive/*17402*-roundup-causes-non-alcoholic-fatty-liver-disease-at-very-low-doses
125   http://www.naturalnews.com/*037249*_GMO_study_cancer_tumors_organ_damage.html
126   http://www.slideshare.net/digitalreporter/the-documented-health-risks-of-genetical-ly-engineered-foods-long-version slide *30* slide *49*
127   https://www.academia.edu/*542384*/A_Review_on_Impacts_of_Genetically_Modified_Food_on_Human_Health
128   http://www.slideshare.net/digitalreporter/the-documented-health-risks-of-genetical-ly-engineered-foods-long-version slide *38*
129   www.bing.com/search?pc=COSP&ptag=D*031616*-A6EC39D5B4CB*74905*A0F&form=CONBDF&conlogo=CT*3332023*&q=collective+evolution+*10*+scientific+studies+proving+gmos+can+be+harmful+to+human+health
130   http://www.slideshare.net/digitalreporter/the-documented-health-risks-of-genetical-ly-engineered-foods-long-version slide *115*
131   www.bing.com/search?pc=COSP&ptag=D*031616*-A6EC39D5B4CB*74905*A0F&form=CONBDF&conlogo=CT*3332023*&q=collective+evolution+*10*+scientific+studies+proving+gmos+can+be+harmful+to+human+health
132   *Genetic Roulette, The Gamble Of Our Lives Movie*
133   http://enveurope.springeropen.com/articles/*10.1186/2190-4715-23-10*
134   http://gmwatch.org/news/latest-news/*17483 2/27/17* Published in GM Watch, **The 750 studies that GMO regulatory bodies often ignore**.
135   Robyn O'Brien Facebook posting *2/27/17*
136   http://www.gmwatch.org/videos/food-safety-videos/*13209*-dr-don-huber-warns-of-a-new-pathogen-linked-with-roundup-ready-gmo-corn

137   www.bing.com/search?pc=COSP&ptag=D031616-A6EC39D5B4CB74905A0F&form=C ONBDF&conlogo=CT3332023&q=collective+evolution+10+scientific+studies+prov- ing+gmos+can+be+harmful+to+human+health

138   www.bing.com/search?pc=COSP&ptag=D031616-A6EC39D5B4CB74905A0F&form=C ONBDF&conlogo=CT3332023&q=collective+evolution+10+scientific+studies+prov- ing+gmos+can+be+harmful+to+human+health

139   http://gmwatch.org/news/latest-news/17456

140   *Genetic Roulette, The Gamble Of Our Lives Movie*

141   http://www.slideshare.net/digitalreporter/the-documented-health-risks-of-genetical- ly-engineered-foods-long-version slide *36*

142   https://www.youtube.com/watch?v=lZ2gCx3WFSo

143   http://althealthworks.com/10609/monsanto-losing-tens-of-millions-on-in-india-as- government-farmers-drop-gmo-cotton/

144   http://www.slideshare.net/digitalreporter/the-documented-health-risks-of-genetical- ly-engineered-foods-long-version slide *106*

145   https://s3-us-west-1.amazonaws.com/www.agrian.com/pdfs/Liberty_Herbicide_ (032806notif041807)_Label.pdf

146   http://www.slideshare.net/digitalreporter/the-documented-health-risks-of-genetical- ly-engineered-foods-long-version slide *51*

147   http://gmwatch.org/latest-listing/1-news-items/6416-mortality-in-sheep-flocks-after- grazing-on-bt-cotton-fields-warangal-district-andhra-pradesh-2942006

148   http://www.isis.org.uk/CAGMMAD.php

149   http://www.slideshare.net/digitalreporter/the-documented-health-risks-of-genetical- ly-engineered-foods-long-version slide *88*

150   www.bing.com/search?pc=COSP&ptag=D031616-A6EC39D5B4CB74905A0F&form=C ONBDF&conlogo=CT3332023&q=collective+evolution+10+scientific+studies+prov- ing+gmos+can+be+harmful+to+human+health

151   http://www.organic-systems.org/journal/81/8106.pdf

152   http://www.ijbs.com/v05p0706.htm

153   http://www.momsacrossamerica.com/zenhoneycutt/mom_s_testimonials

154   Arpad Pusztai, "Can science give us the tools for recognizing possible health risks of GM food," *Nutrition and Health*, 2002, Vol 16 Pp 73-84; Stanley W. B. Ewen and Arpad Pusztai, "Effect of diets containing genetically modified potatoes expressing Galanthus nivalis lectin on rat small intestine," Lancet, 1999 Oct 16; 354 (9187): 1353-4; and Arpad Pusztai, "Facts Behind the GM Pea Controversy: Epigenetics, Transgenic Plants & Risk Assessment," Proceedings of the Conference, December 1st 2005 (Frankfurtam Main, Germany: Literaturhaus, 2005)

155   http://www.economist.com/news/europe/21639578-eu-lifts-its-ban-gm-crops-gen- tly-modified

156   http://www.monsanto.com/improvingagriculture/pages/feeding-the-world.aspx

157   http://farmwars.info/?p=10046

158   http://gmoinside.org/great-food-war-will-won-independent-science-news/

159   Jeffry Smith statement in *Genetic Roulette, The Gamble Of Our Lives Movie*

160   http://www.realfarmacy.com/400-companies-no-gmos/
161   http://www.westonaprice.org/health-topics/how-to-avoid-genetically-modi-fied-foods/
162   I have a copy of an article from AgriNews saved from August 20, 2016 that is no longer available on the internet. The name of the article is "Millennials want organic foods, transparency."
163   http://www.ecowatch.com/regenerative-farming-ocean-acidification-2175984298.html?page=1

Roundup Ready© is a trademark of **Monsanto Company.**
Roundup® **is** a trademark of **Monsanto Company**
Liberty Glusofinate© is a trademark by **Bayer**
Additional reading
http://www.collective-evolution.com/2014/04/08/10-scientific-studies-proving-gmos-can-be-harmful-to-human-health/

CHAPTER 7 TOXINS IN OUR PROCESSED FOOD AND FAST FOOD

165   https://www.youtube.com/watch?v=bpOHUQO0ulE
166   http://www.drfranklipman.com/no-more-msg-the-dangerous-food-additive-you-must-live-without/
167   http://www.hungryforchange.tv/article/sneaky-names-for-msg-check-your-labels
168   http://articles.mercola.com/sites/articles/archive/2014/02/12/9-dangers-pro-cessed-foods.aspx#!
169   http://newsletters.newsmax.com/blaylock/issues/heal0117/blaylock_heal0117_151.pdf
170   https://authoritynutrition.com/9-ways-that-processed-foods-are-killing-people/
171
172   http://www.nhs.uk/Livewell/Goodfood/Pages/what-are-processed-foods.aspx
173   " https://www.nih.gov/news-events/nih-research-matters/food-additives-pro-mote-inflammation-colon-cancer-mice
174   http://www.nytimes.com/2013/02/24/magazine/the-extraordinary-science-of-junk-food.html?emc=eta1
175   http://sahm.org/health-fitness/your-kids-become-what-you-feed-them-7-dangers-of-fast-food/
176   http://positivemed.com/2013/04/20/10-disgusting-facts-about-fast-food/
177   https://www.umc.edu/News_and_Publications/Press_Release/2013-10-02-01_Chick-en_nugget_autopsy_finds_meat_bone_connective_tissue_fat_and_poor_health_implications.aspx
178   http://whatsonmyfood.org/food.jsp?food=PO
179   http://www.coconutclubvacations.net/organic-fast-food-restaurant-miami-florida/
Dr. Frank Lipman MD and Dr. Joseph Mercola quotes used with permission

CHAPTER 8 SUGAR MAKES US SICK

[181] http://drhyman.com/blog/2014/03/06/top-10-big-ideas-detox-sugar/

[182] Dr. Mark Hyman Explains Sugar Addiction on The View http://drhyman.com/blog/2014/03/03/dr-mark-hyman-explains-sugar-addiction-view/

[183] http://www.veteranstoday.com/2016/04/23/fructose-alters-hundreds-of-brain-genes-leads-to-wide-range-of-diseases/

[184] Dr. Mark Hyman Explains Sugar Addiction on The View http://drhyman.com/blog/2014/03/03/dr-mark-hyman-explains-sugar-addiction-view/

[185] http://drhyman.com/blog/2014/03/06/top-10-big-ideas-detox-sugar/

[186] http://www.nytimes.com/2016/12/30/opinion/a-month-without-sugar.html?emc=edit_ty_20170102&nl=opinion-today&nlid=14230857&te=1

[187] http://www.nytimes.com/2016/12/30/opinion/a-month-without-sugar.html?emc=edit_ty_20170102&nl=opinion-today&nlid=14230857&te=1

[188] http://www.nytimes.com/2016/12/30/opinion/a-month-without-sugar.html?emc=edit_ty_20170102&nl=opinion-today&nlid=14230857&te=1

[189] https://www.youtube.com/watch?v=puTQuAYvfWo JJ Virgin Simple Sugar Swaps UTube

[190] https://iquitsugar.com/5-simple-steps-to-jerfing/

[191] https://seancroxton.leadpages.co/jerf-cookbook/

[192] http://www.huffingtonpost.com/lorie-eber/nutrition-keep-it-simple-stupid_b_8693260.html

[193] http://jjvirgin.com/sugar-swaps/

CHAPTER 9 THE PERILS OF DRINKING SODA

[195] https://www.hsph.harvard.edu/nutritionsource/healthy-drinks/soft-drinks-and-disease/

[196] https://theconsciouslife.com/top-10-inflammatory-foods-to-avoid.htm

[197] htthttps://theconsciouslife.com/top-10-inflammatory-foods-to-avoid.htm p://www.medicaldaily.com/pulse/soft-drink-dangers-8-ways-soda-negatively-affects-your-health-319054

[198] https://www.hsph.harvard.edu/nutritionsource/sugary-drinks-fact-sheet/

[199] http://www.medicaldaily.com/pulse/soft-drink-dangers-8-ways-soda-negatively-affects-your-health-319054

[200] http://www.trueactivist.com/what-happens-to-our-body-after-drinking-coca-cola/

[201] http://www.cbsnews.com/news/caramel-coloring-chemical-linked-to-cancer-found-in-too-high-levels-in-some-colas/

[202] http://theequalizerfcw.blogspot.com/2009/06/how-much-sugar-in-20-ounce-coke-16.html

[203] http://www.eatingwell.com/nutrition_health/bone_health/can_drinking_seltzers_sodas_or_other_carbonated_drinks_harm_bones

[204] https://www.fatsecret.com/calories-nutrition/generic/soda

205 tp://www.michaelsinkindds.com/blog/tag/soda-tooth-enamel/
206 wrap girl with Alex sanguine

CHAPTER 10 CANNED GOODS

208 Deanna Minich, Ph.D. from a posting on Facebook *11/22/2016*
209 http://www.ewg.org/research/bpa-canned-food/health-hazards-bpa
210 http://www.ewg.org/research/bpa-canned-food/recommendations

CHAPTER 11 SOY

212 http://www.doctoroz.com/article/soy-good-bad-and-best
213 https://www.scientificamerican.com/article/soybean-fertility-hormone-isofla-vones-genistein/
214 https://authoritynutrition.com/is-soy-bad-for-you-or-good/
215 http://www.nytimes.com/*2016/12/20*/business/paraquat-weed-killer-pesticide.html?emc=eta*1*&_r=*0*
216 http://www.huffingtonpost.com/dr-mercola/soy-health_b_*1822466*.html
217 January *2017* Blaylock Wellness Report http://newsletters.newsmax.com/blaylock/issues/heal*0117*/blaylock_heal*0117_151*.pdf

CHAPTER 12 DAIRY

219 https://authoritynutrition.com/is-dairy-bad-or-good/
220 http://www.eatwild.com/healthbenefits.htm
221 http://www.eatwild.com/healthbenefits.htm
222 http://www.realmilk.com/safety/fresh-unprocessed-raw-whole-milk/
223 http://articles.mercola.com/sites/articles/archive/*2016/05/02*/full-fat-dairy-lowers-diabetes-risk.aspx
224 https://chriskresser.com/still-think-low-fat-dairy-is-the-healthy-choice-think-again/
225 http://www.probioticscenter.org/fermented-milk-products/
226 http://www.reuters.com/article/us-milk-grass-fed-cows-idUSTRE*64R5GY20100528*
227 http://www.whfoods.com/genpage.php?tname=foodspice&dbid=*130*
228 https://saveourbones.com/osteoporosis-milk-myth/
229 https://saveourbones.com/osteoporosis-milk-myth/
230 https://saveourbones.com/osteoporosis-milk-myth/
231 http://www.cancer.org/cancer/cancercauses/othercarcinogens/athome/recombi-nant-bovine-growth-hormone
232 http://www.shirleys-wellness-cafe.com/NaturalFood/Bgh
233 http://health.howstuffworks.com/wellness/food-nutrition/facts/is-milk-good-for-you.htm
234 http://butterbeliever.com/fat-free-dairy-skim-milk-secrets/

[235] , http://livingtraditionally.com/*6*-secrets-you-dont-know-about-skim-milk/
[236] http://butterbeliever.com/fat-free-dairy-skim-milk-secrets/
[237] http://www.latimes.com/food/dailydish/la-dd-cheese-addictive-drugs-*20151022*-story.html
[238] http://www.globalhealingcenter.com/natural-health/dangers-of-cows-milk/

CHAPTER 13 SENSITIVITIES

[240] http://www.allergysolutionsofindiana.com/allergies.cfm
[241] http://www.canadianliving.com/health/nutrition/article/food-intolerance-vs-food-allergy-vs-food-sensitivity-what-s-the-difference
[242] https://robynobrien.com/protecting-children-from-food-allergies-food-sensitivities/
[243] http://drjockers.com/food-sensitivity-testing-cyrex-comprehensive/
[244] http://drjockers.com/food-sensitivity-testing-cyrex-comprehensive/
[245] http://thedr.com/wp-content/uploads/*2016/06*/The-Conundrum-of-GS-*070716*.pdf
[246] https://draxe.com/search-results/?cx=*010110460513198589347*%3A10dblys_dma&cof=FORID%3A9%3BNB%3A1&ie=UTF-*8*&q=symptoms+of+gluten+sensitivity

Dr. Josh Axe, DC CNX has several blogs on his website that will enlighten you about gluten and about sensitivities. I recommend you read his book, *Eat Dirt: Why Leaky Gut May Be the Root Cause of Your Health Problems and 5 Surprising Steps to Cure It* Harper Wave; 1 edition (March 29, 2016) available on Amazon

Dr. Axe comments used with approval.

Dr. David Jockers comments used with approval.

Dr. Tom O'Bryan now teaches about Gluten sensitivity at the Institute for Functional Medicine. For more information please see other blogs on his website, thedr.com. I also recommend you read his book. *The Autoimmune Fix* Rodale Books; 1 edition (September 20, 2016) available on Amazon all about autoimmune disease.

Follow Robyn O'Brien on Facebook. She became a food advocate because she wanted to protect her children. Her work is amazing and well worth following. She also has an informative website.

CHAPTER 14 FACTORY FARMED MEAT, CHICKEN AND FISH AND GOOD ALTERNATIVES

[248] https://www.paleotreats.com/blogs/paleo-desserts-and-paleo-recipes/whats-the-deal-with-grass-fed-beef
[249] http://drhyman.com/blog/*2014/11/07*/pegan-paleo-vegan/
[250] https: http://drhyman.com/blog/*2014/11/07*/pegan-paleo-vegan/ //www.ams.usda.gov/sites/default/files/media/Organic%20Livestock%20Requirements.pdf
[251] http://www.americangrassfed.org/
[252] http://www.marksdailyapple.com/where-to-buy-grass-fed-beef/
[253] http://grasslandbeef.com/shipping-returns

254 https://www.paleotreats.com/blogs/paleo-desserts-and-paleo-recipes/whats-the-deal-with-grass-fed-beef
255 http://paleoleap.com/importance-of-grass-fed-meat/
256 https://www.bewell.com/blog/meat-smarts-3-ways-get-healthy/
257 https://foodrevolution.org/blog/the-truth-about-grassfed-beef/
258 http://www.wholefoodsmarket.com/blog/whole-story/5-step-chicken-what%E2%80%99s-number
259 http://www.whfoods.com/genpage.php?tname=foodspice&dbid=116
260 http://www.takepart.com/article/2013/04/22/eat-more-lamb
261 http://www.takepart.com/article/2013/04/22/eat-more-lamb
262 http://medical-dictionary.thefreedictionary.com/Heritage+Pork
263 https://draxe.com/the-dangers-of-farmed-fish/
264 https://draxe.com/the-dangers-of-farmed-fish/
265 http://www.ewg.org/research/ewgs-good-seafood-guide
Dr. Axe comments used with approval
Dr. Blum's comments used with permission.

CHAPTER 15 GOOD AND BAD COOKING OILS

267 https://www.nytimes.com/2016/09/13/well/eat/how-the-sugar-industry-shifted-blame-to-fat.html?_r=0
268 http://drhyman.com/blog/2013/11/26/fat-make-fat/
269 ://drhyman.com/blog/2013/11/26/fat-make-fat/
270 https://draxe.com/canola-oil-gm/
271 http https://draxe.com/canola-oil-gm/
    https://en.wikipedia.org/wiki/Trans_fat
272 Dr. Susan Blum, email 1/27/17
273 http://foodidentitytheft.com/trying-to-avoid-almonds-that-are-gassed-heres-a-little-guide/
274 https://www.oliveoiltimes.com/olive-oil-business/north-america/california-ap-proves-olive-oil-standards/41296

275 Additional Reading
    What makes avocado oil so healthy?
    http://www.marksdailyapple.com/whats-so-healthy-about-avocado-oil/
    To check out your brand of Almonds, read this article:
    http://foodidentitytheft.com/trying-to-avoid-almonds-that-are-gassed-heres-a-little-guide/

CHAPTER 16 COSMETICS

[277] http://www.safecosmetics.org/get-the-facts/regulations/us-laws/#sthash.8S1kSP1H.dpuf

[278] http://www.takepart.com/article/*2013/10/29*/toxic-chemicals-in-cosmetics Linda Sharps

[279] http://www.takepart.com/article/*2013/10/29*/toxic-chemicals-in-cosmetics

[280] http://www.takepart.com/article/*2013/10/29*/toxic-chemicals-in-cosmetics

[281] http://www.takepart.com/article/*2013/10/29*/toxic-chemicals-in-cosmetics

[282] http://organicbeautytalk.com/ingredients-to-avoid/

[283] http://organicbeautytalk.com/ingredients-to-avoid/
http://www.pureskincare.co.za/pages/cosmetic-ingredients-to-avoid
http://www.glowingorchid.com/ingredients-we-avoid--why.html

[284] http://www.ewg.org/skindeep/search.php?ewg_verified=products

[285] http://www.ewg.org/research/teen-girls-body-burden-hormone-altering-cosmetics-chemicals/cosmetics-chemicals-concern

[286] http://www.ewg.org/research/teen-girls-body-burden-hormone-altering-cosmetics-chemicals/teens-are-vulnerable

[287] http://soapwallakitchen.com/pages/story

[288] http://www.drfranklipman.com/fragrance-stinks-*4*-reasons-to-stop-using-scented-products/

[289] http://www.drfranklipman.com/fragrance-stinks-*4*-reasons-to-stop-using-scented-products/
https://dash.harvard.edu/bitstream/handle/*1/8965615*/Daum*06*.html?sequence=*2*
http://www.goodguide.com/
http://www.safecosmetics.org/safe-cosmetics-companies/

[290] http://www.ewg.org/research/nailed

[291] https://www.rei.com/learn/expert-advice/sunscreen.html

[292] https://www.truthinaging.com/review/ewgs-picks-for-best-sunscreens-and-moisturizers-with-spf

[293] http://foodbabe.com/*2013/05/05*/what-you-need-to-know-before-you-ever-buy-sunscreen-again/

[294] http://shop.suzycohen.com/collections/all/products/catalase
Additional reading
http://www.naturalcosmeticnews.com/toxic-products/list-of-*15*-toxic-chemicals-to-avoid-in-personal-care-products/

CHAPTER 17 DRINKING WATER

[296] The Food Revolution Network, The Truth about Water and what you need to know to be safe.

[297] The Food Revolution Network, The Truth about Water and what you need to know to be safe.

298   Benefits of Lemon Water: Detox Your Body and Skin Dr. Axe https://draxe.com/bene-fits-of-lemon-water/

299   http://www.ewg.org/tap-water/reportfindings.php

300   , http://www.ewg.org/enviroblog/2016/12/reversal-epa-confirms-fracking-pol-lutes-drinking-water

301   http://www.naturalnews.com/025993.html

302   https://draxe.com/tap-water-toxicity/

303   https://draxe.com/tap-water-toxicity/

304   https://draxe.com/tap-water-toxicity/

305   https://draxe.com/estrogen-epidemic-whats-in-your-water/

306   http://www.ewg.org/research/healthy-home-tips/tip-7-filter-your-tap-water

307   https://draxe.com/estrogen-epidemic-whats-in-your-water/

308   https://draxe.com/estrogen-epidemic-whats-in-your-water/

309   https://draxe.com/estrogen-epidemic-whats-in-your-water/
       http://www.drweil.com/health-wellness/balanced-living/healthy-home/does-alkaline-water-promote-health/
       Dr. Frank Lipman's comments used with permission.

ADDITIONAL RESOURCES

http://static.ewg.org/reports/2010/bottledwater2010/pdf/2011-bottledwater-scorecard-report.pdf?_ga=1.132210060.387560268.1474156772 Lists a grade on many bottled waters. More than 50% of the waters tested on the market failed.

http://www.ewg.org/research/bottled-water-quality-investigation/test-results-chemicals-bottled-water

http://www.ewg.org/research/bottled-water-quality-investigation

https://www.nrdc.org/sites/default/files/bottled-water-pure-drink-or-pure-hype-report.pdf

http://www.waterfiltercomparisons.com/countertop-faucet-water-filters-reviews/#start_compare

http://www.ewg.org/research/ewgs-water-filter-buying-guide?system_type=Under-Sink&technology=&contamcode=&submit_ty_1=Search

https://www.purewatersystems.com/index.php

A much more expensive system that claims to remove all of the toxins in your water.

http://www.nsf.org/

http://www.ewg.org/research/healthy-home-tips/tip-7-filter-your-tap-water

310

311

Dr. Axes comments, used with permission
Ocean Robbins comments used with permission

CHAPTER 18 DRUGS

[312] https://draxe.com/an-aspirin-a-day-causes-more-harm-than-good/

[313] http://www.mayoclinic.org/diseases-conditions/heart-disease/in-depth/daily-aspi-rin-therapy/ART-20046797?pg=2

[314] http://www.mayoclinic.org/diseases-conditions/heart-disease/in-depth/daily-aspi-rin-therapy/ART-20046797

[315] https://draxe.com/an-aspirin-a-day-causes-more-harm-than-good/

[316] https://draxe.com/an-aspirin-a-day-causes-more-harm-than-good/

[317] http://www.everydayhealth.com/drugs/naproxen

[318] https://www.davidwolfe.com/over-counter-drug-1-cause-liver-failure/

[319] http://galacticconnection.com/curcumin-reduces-symptoms-of-anxiety-and-depres-sion-even-in-people-with-major-depression/

[320] https://authoritynutrition.com/top-10-evidence-based-health-benefits-of-turmeric/

[321] http://dailynaturalremedies.com/10-health-benefits-of-ginger/10/

[322] http://naturalbloodthinners.org/ginger-blood-thinner-properties/

[323] http://www.collective-evolution.com/2013/08/09/the-dangers-in-regularly-taking-as-pirin-or-ibuprofen/

[324] http://www.collective-evolution.com/2013/08/09/the-dangers-in-regularly-taking-as-pirin-or-ibuprofen/

[325] http://suzycohen.com/articles/antibiotics-are-stupid-its-up-to-you-to-be-smart/

[326] http://suzycohen.com/articles/antibiotics-are-stupid-its-up-to-you-to-be-smart/

[327] http://suzycohen.com/articles/antibiotics-are-stupid-its-up-to-you-to-be-smart/

[328] http://suzycohen.com/articles/natural-alternatives-to-antibiotics-2/

[329] http://avivaromm.com/how-7-top-herbalists-and-doctors-fight-the-flu/
https://draxe.com/8-natural-allergy-relief-remedy

[330]

[331] http://www.health.harvard.edu/blog/common-anticholiner-gic-drugs-like-benadryl-linked-increased-dementia-risk-201501287667
https://draxe.com/8-natural-allergy-relief-remedies/

[332]

[333] https://draxe.com/stinging-nettle/

[334] http://suzycohen.com/articles/ppi_acid_blockers_risk_stroke/#.WEBr_ycECqY.mailto

[335] http://suzycohen.com/articles/ppi_acid_blockers_risk_stroke/#.WEBr_ycECqY.mailto

[336] http://suzycohen.com/articles/5-minute-health-hacks/?inf_contact_key=6e27d603b-8becafe70a32b3bdfd7d4666c58e0af3b580909f7fe3cefd283c78b

[337] http://www.womansmagazine.net/petroleum-jelly-side-effects-and-dangers.html

[338] http://www.womansmagazine.net/petroleum-jelly-side-effects-and-dangers.html

[339] http://www.greenenvee.com/the-dangers-of-petroleum-jelly/

[340] http://shop.themiraclesalve.com/Super-PAV-Oil-2-floz-Bottle-po4ptr.htm

[341] http://www.activationproducts.com/product-category/ease/

342 https://www.rockymountainoils.com/?utm_source=bing&utm_medium=cpc&utm_
      campaign=WP%20-%20Brand&utm_term=rocky%20mountain%20essential%20
      oils&utm_content=Rocky%20Mountain%20Oils
343 http://www.life.ca/naturallife/0808/asknl.htm
      Suzy Cohen's comments used with permission
      Dr. Josh Axe's comments used with permission

ADDITIONAL READING

https://www.bewell.com/blog/problem-nsaids-yes-mean-advil/
http://avivaromm.com/flu-everything-to-know/
http://avivaromm.com/flu-season-hits-hard-again/
http://www.livestrong.com/article/226763-side-effects-of-petrolatum/

CHAPTER 19 CLEANING SUPPLIES

345 http://www.ewg.org/guides/cleaners/content/spring_2016_update
346 http://www.ewg.org/guides/cleaners/content/spring_2016_update
347 http://www.ewg.org/guides/cleaners/content/spring_2016_update
348 http://www.ewg.org/guides/cleaners/content/spring_2016_update

CHAPTER 20 TOXIC METALS

350 http://www.naturalnews.com/055962_heavy_metals_detoxify_Wendy_Myers.html
351 http://articles.mercola.com/sites/articles/archive/2008/07/22/toxic-metals-the-rea-
      son-you-still-feel-sick.aspx#!,

CHAPTER 21 TOXINS IN YOUR KITCHEN- POTS AND PANS, UTENSILS, AND FOOD STORAGE

353 https://whatscookingamerica.net/LindaPosch/ToxicCookware.htm
354 https://whatscookingamerica.net/LindaPosch/ToxicCookware.htm
355 https://www.bewell.com/blog/which-is-the-safest-cookware/
356 https://wellnessmama.com/5148/safest-cookware-options/
357 http://www.ewg.org/research/ewgs-water-week/mad-monday-what-you-dont-know-
      may-hurt-you
358 http://www.mommypotamus.com/diy-reusable-food-wrap/
359 http://www.care2.com/greenliving/vinegar-kills-bacteria-mold-germs.html
360 http://www.using-hydrogen-peroxide.com/home-uses-for-hydrogen-peroxide.html

INTRODUCTION – PART 5 TOXIC MINDS/TOXIC BODY

362 These *12* Primary Elements are synthesized from many and diverse sources. Too many to reference here.

CHAPTER 22 TOXIC STRESS

364 http://www.healthline.com/health/stress/effects-on-body
365 http://www.jakeshealthsolutions.com/the-negative-effects-of-stress-*519*
366 http://www.huffingtonpost.com/*2013/02/04*/stress-health-effects-cancer-immune-system_n_*2599551*.html?slideshow=true#gallery/*278283/0*
367 *ANTs* is a term coined by Daniel Amen, MD and it stands for Anxious Negative Thoughts
368 http://www.medscape.com/viewarticle/*823339*
369 http://blogs.webmd.com/sleep-disorders/*2010/07*/dreams-nightmares-and-stress.html
370 http://www.calmclinic.com/anxiety/symptoms/hair-loss
371 https://www.drweil.com/health-wellness/body-mind-spirit/stress-anxiety/breathing-three-exercises/
372 www.changeyourenergy.com/shop/productdetail.aspx?id=*609*
373 https://www.facebook.com/walkwaytowellness/

CHAPTER 23 TOXIC RELATIONSHIPS

375 http://elitedaily.com/dating/*13*-signs-youre-toxic-relationship-ruining-life/*966801*/
376 http://www.wikihow.com/Recognize-a-Toxic-Friend
377 http://kriscarr.com/blog/how-to-identify-and-release-toxic-relationships/

CHAPTER 24 "ANTS"

379 A term coined by Daniel Amen, MD. *ANTs*- Anxious Negative Thoughts,
380 http://www.amenclinics.com/cybcyb/*12*-prescriptions-for-creating-a-brain-healthy-life/
381 Already Always Listening™ Landmark Worldwide, LLC. http://www.trademarkia.com/map/already-always-listening-*78113582*.html." In my bantering with a former business partner who went through Lifespring courses, it became our term for being stuck in our own "known truth," even though this "truth" may or may not have been true.
382 http://msaprilshowers.com/mind/*9*-types-of-automatic-negative-thoughts-by-dr-d-g-amen/
383 http://danielamenmd.com/*3*-quick-steps-to-stop-negative-thinking-now/

384 http://www.amenclinics.com/blog/learn-anteaters-reduce-stress-anxiety/?utm_
medium=email&_hsenc=p2ANqtz-9Fsq7JG62ISIcOpwNJ9KZ3Ux18eW2AUh9Y-
H0pGNzVGo59T1X-aihk9iHsICAETW8tRX8RJjVopbeRKdM9WTZMS7G1rTw&_
hsmi=39132872&utm_content=39132871&utm_source=hs_email&hsCtaTrack-
ing=89cd75a1-3dd1-4fb0-aa77-ff6289262174%7Cb7099480-e48f-4b3e-b60e-f7a-
f78a4337e
385 http://www.pacificinstitute.co.uk/solutions/investment-in-excellence/
386 http://juliacameronlive.com/basic-tools/morning-pages/
387 Sedona Mago Retreat
388 Elizabeth Ryder, in a conference call *1/5/2017* "Success Challenge"
389 http://deannaminich.com/

CHAPTER 25 TOXIC LACK OF SLEEP
AND WHAT TO DO ABOUT IT

391 https://www.drweil.com/health-wellness/body-mind-spirit/sleep-issues/an-inter-
view-with-rubin-naiman-phd/
392 https://www.drweil.com/health-wellness/body-mind-spirit/sleep-issues/an-inter-
view-with-rubin-naiman-phd/
393 http://ergonomics.about.com/od/Sleep_And_Ergonomics/a/What-Happens-When-
You-Sleep.htm
394 https://www.sciencedaily.com/releases/2008/09/080902075211.htm
395 https://www.nhlbi.nih.gov/health/health-topics/topics/sdd/why
396 http://www.ecowatch.com/8-ways-to-ensure-a-better-nights-sleep-1891115877.html
397 http://www.bing.com/search?pc=COSP&ptag=D031616-A6EC39D5B4CB74905A0F&fo
rm=CONBDF&conlogo=CT3332023&q=is+lack+of+sleep+a+sign+of+depression
398 https://modernancestor.net/2016/08/11/autoimmune-flares-possible-triggers-solu-
tions/
399 http://www.medicalnewstoday.com/articles/282413.php
400 http://healthysleep.med.harvard.edu/need-sleep/whats-in-it-for-you/mood
401 https://www.hsph.harvard.edu/nutritionsource/sleep/
402 https://en.wikipedia.org/wiki/Microsleep
403 https://www.nhlbi.nih.gov/health/health-topics/topics/sdd/why
404 http://www.cnn.com/2012/10/15/health/sleep-insulin-resistance/index.html
405 http://www.ecowatch.com/8-ways-to-ensure-a-better-nights-sleep-1891115877.html
406 http://www.phoenixhelix.com/2015/01/11/can-skipping-sleep-cause-an-autoim-
mune-flare/
407 http://www.ecowatch.com/8-ways-to-ensure-a-better-nights-sleep-1891115877.html
408 https://www.brainmdhealth.com/blog/do-this-not-that-10-tips-for-a-better-nights-
sleep/
409 http://avivaromm.com/sleep-well-7-natural-tips-for-getting-great-zzzzz/
410 http://www.davidwolfe.com/banana-cinnamon-tea-deep-sleep/

CHAPTER 26 MOVEMENT- REMOVING THE TOXIC SLUDGE

[412] http://www.huffingtonpost.com/*2012/03/23*/exercise-health_n_*1374389*.html?slide-show=true#gallery/*216661/5*

[413] http://www.popsci.com/animals-deep-sea-fisherman-in-russia-tweeting-are-weird-looking

[414] http://www.evolutionhealth.com/rebounder/rebounding-benefits.htm

[415] https://wellnessmama.com/*13915*/rebounding-benefits/

About the Authors

CHERYL MEYER AKA CHERYL M HEALTH MUSE

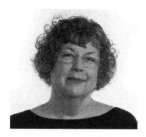 Cheryl is an entrepreneur and Type A personality. For the last *20* years, she has owned a sterling silver jewelry company where she designed jewelry for major retailers. Previously, she was a General Store manager for a major department store where she managed and coached over *200* employees to be their best.

Cheryl is as Integrative Nutrition Health Coach, aka Cheryl M Health Muse. She is a self-published author and an anti-toxin advocate.

Why did she become a health muse? To put it simply, Cheryl got sick, very sick. She had terrible pain and wasn't finding answers. Now on the road to wellness, she w*ants* to share what she has learned to help others.

What can this health muse do for you? Cheryl will inspire you to take charge of your life and reduce your pain. She will help you find the answers you need for wellness. She w*ants* her journey back to wellness to help you in your journey. Cheryl has a mission. She w*ants* to teach you how to live clean and eat clean in a toxic world.

Cheryl is a newly-wed, (at a ripe old age) and married for *2* years to her perfect match in the greater Pasadena, California area.

Cheryl happily reports, "I FEEL GREAT AGAIN, and so can you!"

Cheryl is available for individual and group coaching as well as public speaking and workshops. You can contact her at cherylnhealthmuse@gmail.com and follow her on Facebook as Cherylmhealthmuse.

Want to be the first to know? Follow what she is doing next and stay informed with the latest and the greatest new information. Her newsletters and blogs will be all about living the good life pain-free without toxins and without deprivation.

NICHOLAS PATTON, ILLUSTRATOR

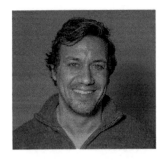

Nick Patton is a multidisciplinary artist living in Portland, OR. He received his BFA in illustration from Columbus College of Art and Design in Columbus, OH and his MFA in Visual Studies from Pacific Northwest College of Art. Nick currently serves as the shop manager for PNCA's sculpture facilities while also completing freelance illustration projects and maintaining a fine art practice that ranges from printmaking to abstract sculpture.

For more information visit www.nickpattonart.com or contact Nick at nick_the_illustrator@yahoo.com

Special thanks to Nick for an outstanding job!!!

Made in the USA
Middletown, DE
17 July 2018